Breathless

Breathless

by
Eric Chason

CIRCLE OF SPIRIT
Chapel Hill, North Carolina

Circle of Spirit Publications
  c/o Drama Circle
P.O. Box 3844
Chapel Hill, NC 27515 USA

Email: info@dramacircle.org
Website: www.circleofspirit.org

Cover design art by David Winsor and Cate Chason. Back cover image taken from the pastel drawing "Breathing Tree" by Cate Chason.

Breathless

19 20 21 22 23 24   10 9 8 7 6 5 4 3 2 1

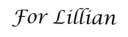

For Lillian

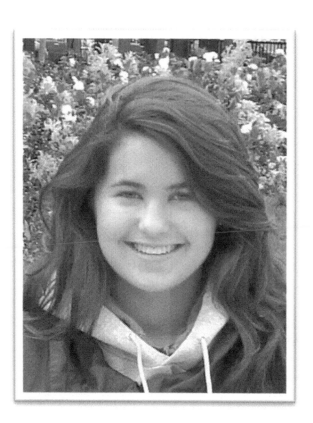

Chapter 1

On the Thursday before Thanksgiving of her freshman year, my daughter Lillian woke up in her dorm room in the middle of the night. She felt terrible. She had been sick all week, had a fever, couldn't breathe, and was worried about all the classes she had missed.

Since September, there had been an H1N1 epidemic at the University of North Carolina and the doctor at the university health services said she was likely to get more symptoms. "Don't come back for a few days," he told her, so she had been riding it out in her room. Her friends had brought her saltines and ginger ale, but she kept feeling worse.

On that Thursday night, her main concern was getting to the bathroom. Like many students, she had her bed lofted up on stilts so that her desk could fit underneath it. She wasn't sure she'd be able to crawl to the far end of the bed and climb the six feet down to the floor.

But she couldn't wait any longer. Forcing herself up onto all fours, she pushed the covers off, then slowly turned around and made her way toward the end. Her muscles burned and her chest felt like there was a huge weight pressing on it. She dragged herself over the railing and down the side, putting one foot on the dresser as she always did, careful not to step on the make-up items she kept there.

The hallway light was painful as she shuffled to the bathroom down the hall. When she got back to her room, the climb back up into bed was too much. Wrapping her bathrobe around her, she lay down on the floor and went to sleep. Her roommate must have walked around her in the morning when she left to go to her classes.

I'd first found out that Lil was getting sick the previous Sunday. It was a bright, autumn afternoon in Rhode Island, leaves falling from the trees as we began the descent into winter. Cate, my wife, was outside in the yard putting her garden to bed for the year. I was sitting in my study going over the remaining lectures for the class that I was teaching that semester. Only one more week to go before the Thanksgiving break.

We were looking forward to our daughters coming home from college for the first time since the school year had started. Already, a small pile of groceries was growing in the kitchen to meet everyone's expectations. Bread crumbs for the sausage stuffing. Marshmallows to be toasted on top of the sweet-potato casserole. Two kinds of cranberry sauce – whole berry and jellied. We had to have an argument every year over which was better.

Around noon, my phone lit up with a text from Lil: "What's the number of the eye doctor down here?"

I looked out the window to see Cate standing next to a bag of leaves in her floppy hat and gardener's gloves, talking on her phone. I walked outside and she held up her hand for me to wait, then filled me in after the call ended.

Lillian had said her head was hurting and she had a shooting pain behind her eyeballs. About two years earlier, she had been diagnosed with Stargardt's disease, a genetic form of macular degeneration that happens when you're young, slowly destroying the central portion of the retina. A black hole was growing in the middle of her vision. It would keep expanding until she was legally blind. The pain she was feeling that weekend had made her terrified that it was suddenly getting worse.

Lil was worried about missing classes and all the work she had, but Cate had told her it was more important to take care of herself. "Get some rest and stay hydrated."

On Monday morning, Lil had called the eye doctor and gotten an appointment for Tuesday. She'd then asked Cate to talk to the disabilities services to arrange for them to take her to the appointment. Cate knew it must be serious if Lil was asking for help.

After seeing the doctor, Lillian called Cate to report on what he said. She was relieved to learn there were no new problems with her eyes. He'd told her that she was probably getting the flu and suggested she go to the university health services, but she was too tired, and it was hard to get there by herself. So she went back to her dorm and said she would go the next day.

Cate begged Lil to let her fly down and help, but Lil wouldn't have it.

"I'm a big girl. If you don't stop talking about coming here, I won't call you anymore."

Cate backed off, but only by making Lil promise to stay in touch.

I kept telling Cate not to worry. "It's just the flu." Like most things, I was sure it would work out.

On Thursday morning, Cate begged her to go back to the doctor but Lil insisted that he had told her not to come back for at least two days.

"He said it was going to get worse," Lil said. "Besides, he didn't do anything. He just told me to take Aleve."

By Friday morning, Cate was frantic. She called her cousin, Melinda, who lives near the university, and asked her to take Lil back to the doctor.

When Melinda got to the dorm, she called from the parking lot to let Lil know she was there. As she waited, a young woman came staggering out of the front door. "Drunk so early in the morning. How sad," Melinda thought. Like Cate, she had been a student at UNC, so it didn't really surprise her.

Until she recognized that it was Lillian. Melinda hurried her into the car then raced over to the health services, where they quickly transferred Lil to the emergency room of the university hospital.

Melinda called Cate to tell her where they were and let her know she would stay with Lil.

Cate called me but I was in the middle of a lecture and didn't take her call. When I got back to her, she started screaming at me. "You need to come home NOW."

She was on the computer trying to buy airline tickets when I arrived. We had already missed one possible flight and she was mad at me because of it. As she looked for others, we agreed that I would stay home to watch the dogs and be there when our other daughter, Hannah, came home on Sunday.

Then the doctor from the emergency room called. "She is having a hard time breathing and is getting very tired," he said. "We want to put her on a ventilator. It would assist her breathing and let her rest."

As a scientist, I am used to understanding data and the natural world. I like to think I'm fairly smart. But in terms of emotional intelligence I can be pretty challenged. I'd been telling Cate that she was overreacting, and now the doctor was patiently explaining the situation to me so I could understand how serious it was. Cate had felt this all along and was frustrated that I didn't get it.

"We'll need to sedate her after we put the tube in," he said. "I asked her who she wants to make decisions for her while she's unconscious and she said that you should."

This was the kick in the head I needed to crack the shell of cluelessness surrounding me.

"I'll do it," I told him and then he let me speak to her. He held the phone to her ear so she could hear.

"Don't be scared," I said. "We're on our way down. We'll be there as soon as we can. We love you."

"I love you too," she said. Then I hung up without thinking, not giving Cate the chance to talk to her.

The doctor told us later that Lil had been very brave when he talked to her about going on the ventilator. "The only time she broke down," he said, "was when she asked, 'Does this mean I can't go home for Thanksgiving?'."

At this point, we could only get a flight as far as Baltimore. Our friend, Pat Lea, was at the rehearsal dinner for her son's wedding (where we were supposed to be that night) and she wanted to help. In between courses, she arranged for a car to pick us up in Baltimore and drive us to Chapel Hill.

We flew into Baltimore around midnight and found the driver holding a sign with our name. He led us to a large Lincoln town car and we sank into the big leather seats in back. As we drove through the black night, I put my head against the door, trying to sleep, but unable to as my thoughts stayed with Lil at the hospital. Cate and I didn't speak to each other at all.

I looked up at the stars as we passed through the invisible countryside of Virginia and North Carolina, on roads we had driven so many times to visit Cate's family. On those trips, we had a van full of summer clothes, bathing suits and beach toys. The girls would pile up towels around themselves, building little nests to hibernate in as they listened to their music or played our one video game. The car was filled with excitement and anticipation, not the hollowness and fear I felt now.

We stopped once for gas around 3 a.m. Leaving the bubble of the car was like a plunge into cold water as we stepped into the night air and the glare of the truck stop. Cate was shivering and I put my arm around her as we went to find the restrooms.

We arrived at the hospital around 5 a.m. on Saturday morning and found our friend, Leslie, there by Lillian's bedside. She had been having a dinner party for her husband's birthday when she learned that Lil was in the hospital. She had come in around midnight and stayed with her all night, not wanting her to be alone.

Chapter 2

From the journal that I started for Lillian to give to her when she got better:

> *Saturday 11/21 – You were in the pediatric intensive care unit (PICU). Kathy Short, the head of respiratory therapy, came in, even though she doesn't normally work on the weekends – she's from Rhode Island originally so she had a special affinity for you. They have put you on a special type of ventilator that is used primarily for burn patients. She's an expert with it and wanted to make sure it was set up correctly.*
>
> *Your sedation isn't too strong and you seem to understand what we are saying, even though you can't respond. It's like talking to someone who is asleep. You take your mother's hand and trace the name "Matt" on it with your fingers. Cate has been talking to him and she tells you he is trying to get down there.*

Lillian's bed was in a small room in the pediatric intensive care unit (PICU). Though she was 18, she was, luckily, considered young enough to be assigned a bed where there were other children. The PICU nurses were warm and caring, accustomed to dealing with premature babies and sick kids, not afraid to let their mothering instincts out.

The sight of Lil in her hospital bed was a father's greatest horror. She was unconscious, lying on her back with her eyes closed. Her small, precious body was pierced by IV lines connected to a stand of pumps that pushed fluids, drugs and antibiotics into her blood stream. She had a breathing tube in her mouth so she couldn't speak to us, even if she weren't sedated. It was hooked up to a ventilator that forced oxygen into her lungs because they were so stiff, she couldn't make them work by herself. The ventilator's sound stood out above all the others in the room, repeating the same pattern over and over, reminding us of the simple act of breathing that we always took for granted. A whoosh of air blowing in, a taka-taka-taka of small pulses to gently force open her airways, then another whoosh of air blowing out.

The cramped room was filled with electronic equipment. Wires from different sensors snaked all over the bed and were collected into a thick bundle near her pillow, then fed over the side of the bed to a rack of monitors. An oxygen sensor attached to her finger glowed red, reminiscent of ET's finger in the movie. Multiple screens kept track of her vital signs, constantly reading out her blood pressure, heart rate, respiration rate and blood-oxygen levels.

These numbers became my lifeline, translating her condition into data, something I could understand. The oxygen level (called her "sats" for "percent saturation") was the most direct indicator of how her lungs were functioning. It had a maximum value of 100 and with the help of the ventilator, the number remained in the low 90s most of the day while she was resting.

Every few hours, a respiratory therapist would come in and, with the nurse's help, suction Lil's lungs to see if they could bring up some of the secretions that were filling them. This was done by lowering another tube through the one that went down her throat and required turning off the ventilator briefly. Each time they did it, her oxygen level dropped from the 90s down into the 70s, then recovered only very slowly. Without the ventilator's support, her lungs quickly filled with fluid, like those of a person who is drowning.

Saturday afternoon - Your X-rays still show some black areas that indicate where the lungs are clear, but there is a lot of white creeping into them, showing where they are filled with fluid. Sometime during the day, one of the nurses tells us they are considering putting you on a machine called ECMO (for extra-corporeal membrane oxygenation). It's basically an artificial lung that puts oxygen directly into your blood and allows your own lungs to rest. However, so far you are still able to get enough oxygen into your lungs with the help of the ventilator.

Lillian's boyfriend, Matt, arrived around 9 p.m. after he managed to catch one of the last flights available during the buildup to the Thanksgiving holiday. I'd told Cate that I didn't know whether this was a good idea, that his family would be upset that he was coming down to North Carolina for his first holiday since starting college. But she said that it was Matt's mother's idea for him to come down and she had even bought him the ticket.

I made a mental note to tell Lil about this. She had told me many times that she didn't think Matt's mother liked her very much.

Although girls' fathers are supposed to dislike their daughter's boyfriends, it was hard to find anything about Matt to disapprove of. He and Lillian had been going out since just before her junior prom, a year and a half earlier. Tall, fair-haired and apple-cheeked, somewhat shy, and polite to a fault, he was literally a Boy Scout, having earned his Eagle Badge a few months earlier. Cate and I were amazed that we'd never heard them utter a harsh word about each other in all the time they'd been together. Unlike most high-school romances, theirs was remarkably free of drama and they often seemed like an old married couple, happy just to hang out together, sitting on the couch and watching movies.

What endeared him to me most was how considerate and protective he was. Before their prom, when everyone was taking pictures outside, he was concerned about whether it was okay for her to take off her sunglasses because of her eye condition. In crowds, he would take her arm as they walked and help her navigate through them. One of her biggest fears in going to college had been wondering who was going to help her find her way around the way Matt had helped her. They had apparently agreed that they weren't going to remain a couple after they went to college, but we knew they still talked to each other often and neither had started a relationship with anyone else.

When he showed up at the door to Lil's room, he had the wide-eyed look of someone out of his element and it made him look even younger than his years.

Cate went up to him right away and steered him through the room and over to Lil's bedside. She gave him Lil's hand and showed him what to watch out for, where the wires and tubes were that he had to be careful of. A quick learner, he was grateful for the orientation and being told how he could act.

Even though Lil was sedated and connected to a dozen machines, Matt didn't skip a beat. He leaned down and spoke into her ear, letting her know he was there.

We could tell immediately that Lil recognized him by the increase in her heartbeat, going up to over 120 per minute. The nurses had told us they wanted her to remain calm, but there was nothing we could do about this. In spite of the drugs, we could see her struggling to force open her reluctant eyelids. After succeeding enough to catch a brief glimpse of him, her lips creased up into a smile around the oxygen tube taped to her mouth. She eventually began to relax as Matt remained sitting next to her, holding her hand and talking to her.

The administrative assistant from the ICU desk came in to ask us who Matt was, reminding us that only family was allowed into her room.

Without hesitation, Cate lied that he was Lil's brother.

The young woman looked at Cate skeptically, but Cate returned her look firmly, making it clear that you didn't want to mess with her about this.

After she left, our nurse went over to Cate and, having seen how Matt talked to her, asked, "Is he really her brother?"

Cate admitted he was Lil's boyfriend, and the nurse gave us a conspiratorial nod that confirmed we were safe. It pretty soon became an open secret and nobody bothered us about it again. We were grateful to be in a hospital down south, where people weren't as strict about the rules as they might be up north.

Cate and I hadn't slept since leaving Rhode Island the night before so we left the hospital around 10 p.m., comforted by knowing that Matt was with Lil. We got a room at the Carolina Inn on campus, the same place where we'd stayed when we first moved Lil to school in August.

Matt came to the Inn around 11:30 and found all the hotel guests on the street and a fire alarm blaring. After the fire department came and the all-clear was sounded, he came up to our room to go to sleep. When he opened the door, he found us still lying there. We had slept right through the fire alarm.

Chapter 3

To understand more about Lillian and how we got to this point, her sixteenth birthday is a good place to start. It was a tricky birthday—too old for kid's games, not quite ready for boy-girl parties. We're not a sweet sixteen type of family, but we still wanted to do something to celebrate it. So Lil was pretty excited when Cate suggested that we take a few of her friends up to Boston for the night.

"Maybe we could spend the night in a hotel?" Lil asked.

When we got the list down to a reasonable size, there were a total of six: four girls, one boyfriend (something new that year) and one male friend to back up the boyfriend. The girls would stay overnight and the boys would just be there for dinner.

This was still too many people to fit into our car. "We'll take the train," Lil suggested. "It'll be fun." So that's how we ended up in the Providence train station with seven teenagers, waiting for the 4:15 to Boston.

We met in the large rotunda, each new arrival greeted with squeals of excitement. The plan was for Cate and me to leave before the train departed so that we could be at the hotel when they got there. I gave them all their tickets and showed them the stairs to the train platform, reminding them to give themselves plenty of time.

"You're sure you know where to go?" I asked for the umpteenth time.

"Yes, Daddy. Don't worry."

"Okay, we'll see you there. Be sure to stay together."

Cate and I climbed into the car and headed away, reassuring ourselves there wasn't much that could go wrong. They didn't have to change trains, and we'd be waiting at the other end.

My cell phone rang when we were outside of Pawtucket heading up I-95, a concrete corridor bordered by old mills. I dug it out of my pants pocket and handed it to Cate. It wasn't Lil, but her ophthalmologist, Dr. Byrne, who wanted to tell us the results of her recent tests. We'd been expecting to hear from him, but I had put it out of my mind. I pulled off at the next exit and found a parking spot in a rundown residential neighborhood.

We locked the car doors and hunched together over the phone as he gave us his report. "I'm pretty certain Lillian has Stargardt's disease," he said. We already knew the significance of the name—we had looked it up on the internet the first time it was mentioned as a possibility. Macular degeneration often causes blindness in the elderly, but Stargardt's occurs in young people. Because he hadn't seen it very often (or maybe it was never), he said we needed to go to Boston to the Massachusetts Eye and Ear Infirmary to confirm it. He would arrange a referral for us.

We thanked him for calling and then sat there, absorbing what we had just heard. This was the most definitive diagnosis we'd received so far. Stargardt's is a progressive condition and her eyesight would get worse until she was legally blind. And once it started, it often worsened rapidly. Her vision at that point was still pretty good, 20/40 with glasses, but it had already been two years since she had first complained that her eyeglasses weren't working. Her optometrist had tried over and over to make her prescription better before he eventually gave up and referred us to the ophthalmologist.

Dr. Byrne had sent us to Rhode Island Hospital to use a newly acquired piece of equipment to measure the responsiveness of her retina. The doctor at the hospital was excited because this was the same piece of equipment they had at Mass. Eye and Ear, and the first one in Rhode Island.

He'd invited me to stay and watch while he conducted the test. He covered one of Lil's eyes with a plastic eyepiece that measured its electrical response while a beam of light was aimed at different parts of her retina.

She sat quietly in the dentist-like chair, trying to keep her head still the way he had asked her. The machine turned the measurements into a contour map of her vision, with the elevations corresponding to the sensitivity in different areas.

I noticed a deep valley in the middle and asked him what that meant. He said that might be where the optic nerve attached to the eye, but he was sure it was normal.

Now, I knew it wasn't. Dr. Byrne had seen the results and said there was clearly a "functional abnormality" in her retina. For the first time, we had to accept that there was something seriously wrong with Lil's eyes.

His words hung like a cloud in the car. How could he have just told us our daughter was going to lose her eyesight? I remember my response in mostly physical terms. My stomach felt empty as the shock set in, a tightening in my chest made it harder to breathe. The deeper feelings of sadness and fear wouldn't come until later. They would sneak up in the darkness, when I lay in bed, listening to the sounds she made in her room as she stayed up late doing her homework. Or, after dropping her off at a friend's house, I'd watch her walk to the front door and disappear inside and I'd wonder how long it would take for her eyesight to grow dim, and how bad it would get.

Cate turned to me and said "It's still her birthday. She doesn't need to hear this today."

"We need to go to Mass. Eye and Ear, anyway, to make sure," I said. I started the car and we got back on the highway.

As I drove, my mind raced with thoughts of what to do. I had read a little about the disease. In a nutshell, a series of reactions in the retina's cells converts light into a chemical signal that's passed onto the optic nerve and fed into the brain. These reactions produce byproducts that have to be flushed away. In the case of Stargardt's, you lose the ability to remove this waste so it builds up and kills the cells. Who did I know at the med school who would know about this? How would I find out what drugs were being developed? What about clinical trials? Why hadn't I taken organic chemistry?

My thoughts were interrupted by the phone ringing again.

"We missed the train."

I was pulled back immediately into full daddy mode.

"WHAT!? You were standing right there. It's so big. It's a train!"

"I know. We were standing around on the platform, talking, and then it started to move. Andrew said 'I think that was our train'."

I could hear my voice starting to rise. "But we have reservations," I said.

Cate looked over at me and mouthed, "Relax."

"I'm turning around—we'll come and get you."

"No. It's okay. There's another train that leaves in 45 minutes. We'll be okay."

This was what was so amazing about having a teenager. One minute she could miss a train that was right in front of her. The next, she had the wherewithal to check the schedule and find another.

"Can you change the reservation to later?" she asked.

I was checkmated. I wanted to be upset, but there really wasn't any reason to. I said, "Sure," and told her we would meet her at the hotel.

"Do you remember where to go?" I asked once more.

"Yes, Daddy," she said. The tone in her voice seemed to ask, "How could you doubt me?", all recent evidence to the contrary.

We finished the drive to Boston through the midafternoon traffic. At the hotel in Copley Place, we checked into our room then went down to the lobby to wait for Lil and her friends.

The gang of seven spilled through the revolving doors, loaded down with backpacks and purses, shoe bags and cosmetics cases. They were laughing and joking as we gave them the key to their room and told them to meet us in half an hour for dinner.

Everybody was hungry by the time we walked across the street to Lil's favorite Italian restaurant. The waiters brought out large platters of pasta and meatballs, salad and garlic bread that we passed around family-style.

While we ate, we told her friends stories about Lil growing up in New Mexico. How when Lil was two years old, Cate and the girls were in Santa Fe and saw a commercial being filmed in the plaza. The director had said that Lil was so beautiful, he wondered if he could use her in the commercial.

We remembered how she used to get horseback riding lessons from a woman who lived way out in the country on a ranch. The two of them would take off riding across the high desert, Lil fearless on a big old horse named Jerry, her little legs spread-eagled across his back.

After cake and presents, we huddled on the busy sidewalk outside the restaurant, discussing what to do next. The two boys danced around as they tried to get out of the way of the purpose-driven Bostonians walking around us, while the girls leaned in, oblivious to the traffic. They decided to go shopping in Copley Place before it closed, so I offered to walk the boys back to the train (and wait to make sure they got on) while Cate went back to our room.

The next morning, Cate and I woke up early and went for a long walk through the empty Sunday-morning streets. A good night's sleep, the early morning air and the memories of the night before gave me a glow of contentment, like a warm blanket enfolding me. Cate held my arm as we strolled down Newbury Street to the public gardens, places we knew and loved from living in nearby Cambridge during graduate school. That had been more than 20 years earlier, and now here we were with a beautiful teenage daughter celebrating her sixteenth birthday. The phone call from the eye doctor wasn't any part of my thoughts. I just felt grateful to know our daughter was happy and that we could do this for her birthday.

When we noticed that a Star Market was open, we stopped and filled up a cart of things to bring back to the girls: juice and chocolate milk, fruit and croissants, mudpacks for their faces and a big helium balloon that said, "Happy Birthday."

We let them sleep as late as we could before going up to their room. The key card didn't work so we had to knock.

"Was everything okay?" I asked as Lil opened the door.

"No problem," she said.

Not an excessively detailed response, but here's what I've pieced together about how they spent the night. They ran around to a bunch of stores until the mall closed, then back to the room for a fashion show with their new purchases. Someone suggested going for a swim, but they didn't know how to get to the pool, so they all got into their bathing suits and jumped into the shower. This was followed by music and dancing until there was a knock on the door.

"Can you open up the door?"

"Oh, my God, Lil! Did you lock it?"

"Who is it?" she'd said as she went up to it and threw the deadbolt.

The other girls had dived into the bed and under the covers.

"It's hotel security. We've had complaints about the noise. Can you open the door?"

"No," Lil had said, "I'm not going to open the door."

"I need to come in."

"That's not going to happen. But we are going to be quiet."

There was a pause, and then he had finally gone away. With the intruder repelled, the other girls had come out of hiding.

"God, I thought it was an ax murderer."

"How did you know what to say? "

"I don't know," Lil said. "But I knew I wasn't opening the door for him."

The other girls told her how amazing it was that she had stayed so cool.

Afterward, they climbed into the beds and watched movies, falling off one-by-one as the night went on.

When we walked in, there were girls scattered all around, some on the bed, others on the floor. Some were still asleep and some were waking up. They had the look of sleepy little kids who had stayed up too late. Groggily, they put themselves back together and made it down to the station in time for the train back home. Lil was the last one left at the Providence station by the time we arrived in the car. As we drove home, she said "That was the best birthday ever."

Two and a half weeks later we were headed back up to Boston to the Massachusetts Eye and Ear Infirmary. They wanted us to be there early in the day, so we left Providence before sunrise. Lil curled up in the back seat and immediately fell asleep while we drove.

MEEI is a large concrete building in a vast hospital complex, right next to Storrow Drive, a major artery going into Boston. Lil held our hands as we navigated through the noisy corridors, first to the registration area and then up to the 6th floor retinology department. Finally we made it to the right waiting room and a young resident introduced herself to us.

Cate and I followed as she led Lil through a battery of tests that lasted all morning and into the afternoon. Lil sat uncomplainingly through each one, trying her best to do what she was asked. Struggling to see the numbers that were hidden in a field of colored bubbles. Sitting gamely in the dark while a bright light was shone in her eyes to measure the thickness of her retina. Not complaining when they repeated the electroretinography test that had already been done in Rhode Island.

It was heartbreaking, not being able to help her when she couldn't see things that appeared so obvious. At 12:30, Cate put her foot down and insisted that Lil take a break to get some lunch. After a quick bite in the hospital cafeteria, we went back for another hour. Finally, the resident pronounced the tests complete and ushered us into an exam room to wait for the results.

The doctor eventually came in, followed by the resident and another intern. He introduced everybody and asked if we needed anything.

Lil was sitting on the edge of the exam table, her legs hanging over and her palms pressed down into the black vinyl cushion top. Every once in a while, she would push down with her hands and lift herself up slightly, suspended by her arms so that her body could swing like a little monkey, using up some of her surplus energy as the resident recited the results of the tests she had performed.

When the resident was done, the doctor pulled his rolling stool up to the table where Lil was perched. He sat down with his head at the same level as hers and he spoke directly to her.

"I'm sorry to be the person to tell you this, but you have Stargardt's disease. It means your eyesight is going to get worse. There's nothing that can be done about it."

While he spoke, she looked at the floor and bit on her bottom lip, gently nodding her head and rocking her body. Then she put her hand on his knee and said, "I understand. It's okay."

He surprised us by turning away from her, trying to hide the tears forming in his eyes. "You know this means you'll probably need to live in a city," he said as he recovered.

Her face brightened a little and she said, "Yeah, that'll be cool."

After the long day, we needed a break before heading home, so we drove across the river into Cambridge, near where Cate and I had lived. We took Lil to the S&S Diner, a place we had often gone to for comfort and good food when we were poor students. The 600-pound gorilla at the table couldn't be ignored, so we talked a little about the hospital and what Lil thought about the doctors. Her assessment: The main doctor, kind. The resident, efficient but a little impersonal. The intern, a geek in high school.

I started to talk about all the wonderful new genetic therapies they were coming up with, but it was clear she didn't want to hear about it so I dropped it.

The main thing she wanted to talk about was her upcoming spring break.

"You know, I'm signed up for driver's ed. But I don't want to spend the whole week in class if I'm not going to be able to drive."

I agreed, but pointed out that her vision was still good. "I think that legally you are allowed to."

"But I wouldn't want to hurt anybody. And what's the point if I'll have to stop soon anyway?"

On the other hand, the allure of driving was pretty strong. Maybe she should try it to see.

"Yeah, don't cancel it yet. Let me think about it."

She fell asleep in the car again on the way home. Her face became angelic in its softness while she dozed, and Cate spent a long time looking back at her while she lay there.

That night, we awoke when we heard her go into the bathroom and start throwing up.

Cate ran to her side and held her while she bent over the toilet. I got a washcloth and soaked it to put on her head.

"I don't know why I'm throwing up," she said after her chest stopped heaving. "I felt fine earlier."

"Maybe it had something to do with the long day you had," Cate said soothingly, rubbing her back.

Lil nodded in agreement, as if this was something she hadn't considered. She came back to bed with us and we all pushed over, making room for her on Cate's side. Cate rolled over towards her, cradling her in her arms for the rest of the night.

The following week I picked her up after school to drive her home. It was a clear early spring day and the forsythia were just starting to come out. There were still two weeks until spring break. I turned onto the street that leads into our neighborhood as she was telling me about her day. I stopped the car because of some children playing in the street.

"Why did you do that?" she asked.

"There are kids there. Do you see them?" I asked.

She turned her head slightly to be able to use her peripheral vision better.

"Oh," she said.

I started driving again and she sat in silence. After that day, we didn't talk again about whether she would get her license.

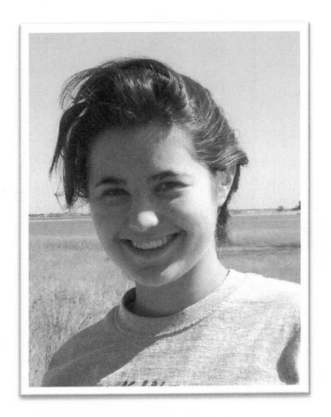

Lillian at the age of 16

Chapter 4

Sunday, 11/22 – You were still in the PICU (pediatric intensive care unit) and on the ventilator that they use for burn patients. We thought that you were making some progress and one of the nurses said she didn't think you would need to go on the ECMO machine. But Kathy Short keeps coming in all weekend to monitor the ventilator and she still seems very concerned.

Not much comes up when they do the suctioning of your lungs but it's very hard on you. It makes you gag and you try to sit up even though you have restraints holding you down. So they start to give you a paralytic to keep your muscles from moving. Because it can be very scary not to be able to move your muscles, they also increase your level of sedation to keep you calm. After this, you can no longer respond to us.

We left Matt sleeping in our room at the inn and got to the hospital right as they were changing from the evening to the morning staff. They asked us to wait until the shift change was over. This was the time that the nurses could speak openly to each other, the night nurse filling in the day nurse on the patient's condition, and they didn't want the families there.

We stood outside the PICU door until they had finished and then they buzzed us in. When we walked into Lil's room I immediately checked the monitors and saw that things hadn't improved overnight. I felt a fleeting sense of disappointment, the kind of emptiness you feel when you've been hoping for something that doesn't happen. I put it aside, telling myself that it just meant that this was going to take awhile, that we were going to have to hope harder, cheer more strongly, stay longer than we had originally thought.

The nurse who took over that morning was friendly and cheerful, constantly in motion, but never hurried. She had three children of her own and she treated Lil as if she were one of them, talking to her, letting her know what she was doing. "Other nurses get burnt out working in the ICU," she told us, "but I still love it."

While she did her many duties—taking blood, cleaning Lil, giving her medication—she asked us to tell her about Lil as a person, not just a patient. She continued to move around the room as we spoke, always keeping her focus on Lil like a watchful mother. Her soft Southern accent was bright and comforting at the same time. She exuded positivity, as if every sentence ended in an exclamation point.

We told her about how Lil was a freshman and wanted to major in drama ("I'll have to take my daughter to see her plays!") and that Cate's family had been in Carolina since the 1600s. ("That explains why she came here!")

Lil lay quietly, her eyes closed, her head turned to one side with the tube of the respirator between her lips, secured in place with tape.

Cate stood next to her and held her head, stroking her full, dark hair. Shoulder-length and wavy, it was the feature that Lil said she loved most about herself.

Cate kissed Lil's forehead, then looked up suddenly. "You washed her hair!" she said.

The nurse smiled and said she had done it that morning before we arrived.

I shook my head in wonder to think how she'd managed it with all the tubes and wires covering the bed.

I asked the nurse whether she knew that Lil had vision problems and she said no. Since Lil had been kept sedated, it wasn't something that was important in her overall condition.

I'd been hesitant to bring it up, because Lil never wanted to be defined by her disability. The average person wouldn't know that she had any problem seeing. She still looked people in the eye when she met them, even though she told me that she couldn't see their faces. People sometimes misunderstood her as being aloof because she didn't greet them, not realizing that she couldn't recognize them. She still had 20/80 vision (with glasses) but it was getting worse, and would continue degenerating.

The nurse listened with sympathy, but not surprise, like someone who is experienced with dealing with bad news. Then she brought the conversation back to an update about Lil's present problems. Overnight, she told us, they had added a muscle paralyzer and increased Lil's sedation. This made her even less able to respond to us than she had been.

"But you should still talk to her," she added. "I've had patients who've gotten better tell me they recognize my voice, even though they were unconscious the whole time."

Cate crouched by Lil's head, talking gently into her ear, stroking her forehead, rubbing her arm while I stood at the foot of the bed. Thoughts drifting, I began to think about how much Lil loved to listen to music and I wondered what had happened to her iPhone. The nurse told me her belongings were in a bag stuffed into the small closet in the corner.

"That's the shawl I just bought her," Cate exclaimed as I took things out of the bag. The shawl was a deep burgundy color, made of soft cashmere. Cate wrapped it around Lil's shoulders as she lay in the bed.

I found the iPhone on the bottom. Sure enough, it had a lot of her favorite music on it. There was even had a playlist labeled 'Songs that make me happy'. As Lil would have said, "How perfect is that?"

I set it up on the pillow next to her head. It could only be heard if you stood right next to it, otherwise it was drowned out by the noise of all the equipment in the room. We took turns standing there, holding her hand and listening.

I hadn't heard her music since she had moved to college and it transported me back in time. Lil would spend hours in front of the computer, sampling music, taking pride in discovering new groups before any of her friends did. Every morning we'd wake to her CD player going off at least half an hour before she could drag herself out of bed for school.

Cate and I would lie in our own bed and listen to her latest obsession, happy to get this window into her life, happy to hear music that we never would have heard otherwise.

It had taken us awhile to find a phone for people with visual impairments. At that time, most phones had tiny screens that Lil couldn't read, but she'd heard that Apple had put accessibility software into their phones so we went to check it out.

Lil explained to the salesperson what her problem was and what she needed. The woman didn't know anything about it at first, but was able to find it easily. They had a mode where you could tap the screen with 3 fingers and the text expanded so that you could read it. It was very intuitive and simple and we were sold.

After Lil got it, she became totally wrapped up in it, to the point where her friends made fun of her for constantly walking around with her head down, looking at the screen as she used one app or another.

Her teacher for the visually impaired had told her that one key to managing in college would be to stay organized, so she learned how to use the scheduler and entered all her important events into it.

In her hospital room now, we were surprised the first time that the phone's alarm went off and said that it was time for her to go to rehearsal for a play she was in. A little chime accompanied by the words "zumba" and "butts, guts and abs" alerted us when it was time for her exercise classes.

We suddenly realized that with her phone, we could contact people at UNC who didn't know she was in the hospital. I didn't really know who her friends were, but I was able to look at her recent text messages to see who she'd been talking to.

On Thursday night, she had written to Z:

> L: Have you ever noticed how when you're sick it's never during a lull like you always have way more shit to do then normal when you're sick
>
> Z: Well obviously. Being sick has to be the all around worst experience possible...
>
> L: Yes it really is. And I don't think I'm ever going to get better
>
> Z: Hey dont say that! Possitive outlook is everything!!! Just think of all the food you'll be eating next week :)
>
> L: Ughhh and all the homework I'll be doing

The same night she wrote to AK:

> L: I am so sick like seriously ill
>
> AK: Dudeee. Are you sure they can't give you meds ?
>
> L: Yeah he said just go home go to sleep and drink fluids
>
> L: And now I'm freaking out because I just have so much work to do
>
> AK: Dude its okay, your teachers have to understand. Just don't stress about it and sleep and get well cuz that's better than half trying to work.
>
> L: Yeah but this is the situation first off my mom wants me to update her but then she freaks out and threatens to come down here so I haven't called her yet and now I'm thinking of all the work I have to do and it's all very time sensitive like I have to go see a three hour long performance TWICE and then I have to write two separate papers on it and all of

the performances are during the rehearsal for my play and apparently my Phil teacher assigned a paper on Wednesday due right after thanksgiving and my english teacher has a paper due Tuesday and when I get back from Thanksgiving. Dram 120 there's a group presentation right after thanksgiving on top of it all I have rehearsal and a final scene for Dram 155 which is basically preparing a play

I hated to see how worried she had been and how she didn't feel she could share it with us. After Friday, the messages started getting more concerned as she stopped answering her phone. On Sunday, her friend D wrote:

> D: Just came and knocked on your door a few times and no one answered… Bit worried. Text me if you get this k?

I called each of them to let them know she was in the hospital and to ask them to pass the information on to her other friends.

Chapter 5

Monday, 11/23 – Although we had thought things were getting better, by Monday it was clear that they weren't improving. So they asked us to meet with the doctors to talk about going on the ECMO machine.

The meeting was led by Dr. Anthony Charles, the surgeon in charge of the program. He explained to us that the ECMO machine wasn't going to heal you, it would just support your body so your lungs could rest and heal themselves—you needed time to overcome the source of the disease and resolve the immune response that your body had made to it. They stressed that there is a window of time during which ECMO is most effective so they don't want to wait too long. If they stick with the ventilator much longer and you don't get better, it won't help to go on ECMO. But it also has significant risks, so they didn't want to put you on it until they were sure that conventional therapies wouldn't work. ECMO couldn't support you forever, and he said that 14 days was a typical period during which you could survive. After that, there would be complications, such as bleeding internally.

Our other daughter, Hannah, had arrived late the night before from Montana, where she was spending her junior year. Fortunately, she'd been able to change the flight that was supposed to take her home to Rhode Island for Thanksgiving.

The four of us had spent the night in two different places. Matt and I went to the Ronald MacDonald House, which provides rooms for families of sick children. They only had space for two, so Hannah and Cate had gone back to the Inn.

They were already in Lil's room when Matt and I arrived by the first shuttle. I gave Hannah a big hug, holding her a long time, burying my face in the long hair she'd grown out since the last time I saw her.

Montana was agreeing with her. She was slender and strong and almost as tall as me now. She was also a little pale.

Cate had taken her up to Lil's bedside but, after standing there for a little while, Hannah had suddenly passed out. Luckily the nurse caught her before her head hit the floor.

Dr. Cairns, the head of the burn unit, came by to talk to us, hanging on to an IV pole as he spoke. He had an interesting demeanor--quiet and reflective one moment, then talkative the next. Cate liked to refer to him as "the cowboy."

I had gotten to know him a little over the weekend when he came to work on Lil's ventilator, a special type used for burn patients. I couldn't imagine the suffering that he's seen working with burn patients, and you could almost feel the weight of it pulling him down.

However, when he found out I was a physicist, he perked up and told me he wanted to stop being a doctor and study high-energy physics (I assumed he was joking). Then he started talking about experiments at the new particle accelerator in CERN and I wasn't so sure.

Lil's numbers looked worse this morning than when we'd left last night, so he wanted us to consider putting her on the ECMO machine. Cairns had been instrumental in bringing ECMO to the hospital because the lung tissue in severely burned patients is too delicate to be stretched by even the most gentle ventilators. In these cases, ECMO is the only remaining option.

It wasn't a light decision. Once Lil was put on it, she couldn't be taken off until her own lungs were better. He told us he would set up a meeting with the head of the program, Dr. Charles, to discuss it further.

Around noon, they brought us into a sterile conference room (appropriate for a hospital, I thought) with plastic chairs, a long Formica table and lights that seemed to belong in an operating room.

Dr. Charles introduced himself and wasted no time lobbying us to put Lillian on ECMO. "Basically," he said, "her lungs are failing and soon, she won't be able to breathe even with the help of the ventilator. If we don't do something soon, it will be too late even for ECMO to help."

It would have been hard not to be convinced by his manner alone—he was very confident, highly energetic and had an infectious laugh. His accent sounded vaguely Jamaican, coming from a mixture of West African and Irish. We learned later that his father, who started out as a pediatrician in Nigeria, had been head of the health services in Africa for Guinness brewery. This had given Dr. Charles the opportunity to go to private school in Ireland for his secondary education.

We were fortunate that UNC even had an ECMO program for adults. In most places it is only used for pediatric patients. This evolved out of studies done in the 1970s, when the technique was first introduced. For adults, the outcome hadn't particularly improved, partially because they would only put the sickest patients on it when it was too late for them to get better.

But one group at the University of Michigan had kept an adult program going and been able to reduce many of the complications. This is where Dr. Charles had studied and he'd been recruited by UNC to develop its adult ECMO program. Only a year and a half old, it had, up to this point, treated just 15 adult patients.

There was still lingering resistance among many doctors to the technique. It required a lot of highly trained staff and a long-term commitment to very ill patients. But a strong case for ECMO was being made in reports from Australia and New Zealand, where they were six months ahead of us in the H1N1 pandemic. Doctors there were finding that it was the only treatment for severely ill patients who couldn't be supported by ventilators alone, with a 75-percent survival rate.

Dr. Cairns spoke after Dr. Charles, but it didn't matter at this point, and I don't even remember what he said. We asked for a few minutes alone and after the doctors left the room, Cate voiced what we all felt: "There doesn't seem to be any choice."

So we called the doctors back into the room and agreed to give our consent to put Lillian on ECMO.

Because of their sense of urgency, we expected it to happen quickly after this. But instead, all the doctors seemed to disappear and we spent the entire day by Lil's bedside waiting, wondering what was going on.

Later that afternoon, the nurse told us about the difficulties they were having. There were four ECMO machines in the hospital but not enough trained staff to run them all. One technician can monitor two machines, but only if they can both be seen continuously, so Lil needed to be in the same place as one of the other ECMO patients. The only available space big enough was in the neurosurgical ICU (NSICU), but the ECMO team was in the surgical unit and Lil was currently in pediatrics. As with any bureaucracy, there were turf wars between departments and it took a full afternoon of negotiations to straighten everything out.

The move didn't occur until that evening but when it happened, it happened quickly. Tubes and wires were disconnected and the machines were replaced with battery-operated units to keep Lil oxygenated and sedated during the move. It was like a parade when they wheeled her bed down the hall with one advance guard clearing the way and seven nurses and technicians surrounding her.

We watched them disappear as they turned the corner into another corridor and then the head nurse directed us to a private conference room where we could wait until the procedure was over.

Dr. Charles came in wearing surgical scrubs and explained what they were going to do. Two tubes, known as canulae, would be inserted into her body. One would go over her right shoulder into her neck to deliver oxygenated blood to the right ventricle of her heart. The blood would be pumped by Lil's heart and sent through her lungs (although they wouldn't be adding any oxygen to it until they got better) and then to the rest of her body. The other canula would be placed in her groin to remove the deoxygenated blood from her veins and send it back to the ECMO machine.

"Putting someone onto the machine is the riskiest part of ECMO," he explained. Their blood has to be made extremely thin to prevent clotting, so any internal bleeding caused by placing the canula would be fatal. The patients are carefully chosen to select only those who can tolerate this phase. When he was done, he asked us if we wanted to go see Lil before he started the operation.

He walked us through the locked NSICU door, past the nurses' station and into a large, triple-width bay surrounded by curtains to screen it off from the hallway. Lil's bed was on the right side of the room surrounded by the same ventilator, monitors and pumps, but with more space than the room in pediatrics. There was a window on the wall behind her, but it was inaccessible because of all the lines, cords and tubes coming out of the wall. Toward the middle of the room was an empty space that was reserved for the ECMO machine.

The other ECMO patient was on the left side of the room. He had a confirmed case of H1N1 and there was a lot of concern about spreading infection, so we each had to put on a surgical mask, gown and gloves whenever we entered the room. The room was strictly divided between his side and ours, as if the room's two occupants were unhappy roommates. We were told to stay away from his bed, and his visitors were kept away from us.

The four of us huddled around Lil as she lay there, the sound of the ventilator beating time as it had in the pediatric unit. Hannah and Matt stood on either side of her, holding her hands. Cate leaned over her head, whispering in her ear and stroking her hair.

When she was done, I kissed Lil's cheek and told her we would be back when they were done. As we walked out of the NSICU, I saw the nurse pull the curtain around Lil's bed so they could get started.

We went back to the conference room to wait. Dr. Charles had promised that he would come in as soon as he was done, but it wouldn't be for a few hours. The hospital had left a cart with snacks and sodas in the room. Nobody was hungry but Cate urged Hannah and Matt to eat something. Cate's cousin, Melinda, arrived after a little while to share the waiting with us.

Around 8 o'clock, we got a call from Mark Perry, one of Lil's drama professors. She was acting in a play he had written and Cate had called him the day before to let him know she wouldn't be at rehearsal tonight. (Her iPhone had told us she was supposed to be there.)

When the cast had found out that Lil was in the hospital, he told Cate, nobody wanted to rehearse. They begged him to call us to find out if they could visit her.

Cate explained that nobody could see Lil tonight. But sensing how scared they were, she told him it was okay to bring them to the room we were waiting in.

All semester, Lil had filled us in about different productions she had auditioned for. It was difficult for a freshman to get a part, but she had a positive attitude, claiming it was all good experience. One role called for someone who played cello and she'd told the director that she could do that.

"Daddy, could you send my cello down?" she'd asked me.

"But you haven't played since you were 12," I said.

"I know, but I think I can remember with a little practice." Luckily the director told her not to bother.

There was nothing better, she told me, than the feeling of being on stage. "It's where I feel most alive."

That wasn't something she got from her parents—neither of us were performers. And she knew how difficult a life it could be, because we have friends who are actors and voice coaches.

But unlike her other work in high school, she had never complained about learning her lines or going to rehearsal. Of course, I worried about how she would be able to pursue it as her eyesight got worse, but she might as well do what she loved while she could.

When she found out that she'd gotten the lead in Mark's play, it was the highlight of her semester.

Matt played for us the voicemail she had left for him when she found out, just three weeks earlier. "Maaaatttttt!!!," her recorded voice screamed. "You have to call me. You'll never guess what happened!"

She had been in many productions in high school, but this was validation that she really had talent. Plus, she was really excited by this play. It was written by one of her professors and told the true story of a young Bahá'í woman named Mona who was persecuted for her religious beliefs after the Iranian revolution. Lil was going to play Mona.

The group of cast members arrived about 20 minutes later, shepherded by Mark. About seven in all, they filled up the room, some using the chairs, the rest perching on tables. The students had the same look that Matt had when he arrived, wide-eyed and totally out of place.

Mark introduced himself and I asked the others to tell me who they were. I recognized some of them from conversations with Lil. Now they had faces to go with their names.

Cate took all the crackers and cookies from the cart and put them on the table. "Please, eat this," she said. Then grabbing Hannah by the arm she said, "I need to take a walk," and dragged her out of the room.

Mark asked how Lil was, and I explained that they were doing a procedure to put her on a machine to breathe for her.

The boys kept looking down, not wanting to make eye contact, the fear and pain evident in their faces.

"But I just saw her last week," said a tall, young, black man."

I recognized him from the freshman orientation we'd attended in August, when Cate had pointed him out to Lil. "You should get to know him. You can tell that he loves his mother."

I made a note to tell Cate that he was there.

One of the girls asked me, "Are you a professor?"

"Yes," I said, "How did you know?"

"Lil found out my father is a professor and she said you are, too. She said to me, 'I bet you're an NPR kid. There are two kinds of kids, those whose parents make them listen to NPR and those who don't'."

Some of the kids smiled even as they continued to look down.

Another girl continued, "Oh, my God, I couldn't believe it the first time I met her. She just plopped down next to me and started talking. About everything ... being a freshman, what's my favorite TV show, what classes I was taking."

Mark added, "When she came to audition, she told me, 'You have got to let me do this play. I just feel so strongly about Mona. It's like I know her'. She would even argue with me about what Mona would say. I told her 'I know people who knew Mona' and she said, 'I don't care. That's not what Mona would say'."

Mark had invited the cast over for dinner to meet his wife Azi. She had actually known Mona when she was younger and wanted to share stories about her with the cast. As Azi told them how Mona and her father were imprisoned for their refusal to give up their religion, Lil started to cry and couldn't stop.

"What meaning does my life have?" she'd sobbed. "Mona gave up everything for her beliefs."

"I didn't really think about what the play meant before that," said one of the boys.

Mark also told us that he had started a Facebook page called "Prayers for Lillian" so that people could share their thoughts and we could share updates about her condition. Azi had put a Bahá'í prayer on the site, and they also put a photo of Mona up on it.

We were shocked when we looked at it later, because we thought it was Lillian, it looked so similar. We understood why Mark had been so excited about her playing the character of Mona.

The cast left after a while, and Cate and Hannah returned.

Finally, Dr. Charles came in to tell us how things went. He collapsed into one of the conference-room chairs, letting his arms and legs spread out as he talked, a big smile on his face. He seemed tired but relieved, so relieved that it made me realize how dangerous the whole procedure had been. But Lil had tolerated it very well and he was pleased with her status.

We were allowed to go in to see her and saw the ECMO machine for the first time. It took up half the room on the left side of the bed. There was a plastic hose carrying bright red blood going into a large tube in her neck. A wide gauze bandage was wrapped around the tube and her forehead to keep the tube from moving. Blood of a darker hue was coming from another tube in her groin that was partially covered by the sheets.

The machine that lay between these two hoses slowly and steadily circulated her blood. A technician sat at the console, constantly monitoring the blood-gas levels to make sure that they were kept within the proper range, changing the flow rate to adjust them if they varied.

I stared at the machine for a long time, mesmerized by its soft but consistent throbbing. Could it be possible that it was doing the job of her own lungs, that her organs could be replaced by this? I couldn't stop watching it, not sure how I could trust it to pump the blood through her body with the tenderness it deserved.

We stayed with her for a while to make sure she was stable, then left for the night.

Chapter 6

Tuesday 11/24 — Matt left on Tuesday morning. He was reluctant to go, but I know he is worried about his mother back in RI. We told him he needed to see his family. Your body started to swell up on Tuesday. We were told that it would get even worse. When you go on ECMO, there is an allergic reaction to all the residual contamination in the tubing that leads to an inflammatory response. This adjustment to the ECMO takes time, so they just let you rest through the day. Later, they will try to start reducing your fluid levels to "dry you out and make you crispy" as Dr. Charles says.

The parents of the other ECMO patient came up to me in the ICU waiting room. The nurses couldn't tell us anything about his case because of privacy rules, but they filled me in. He is 30 years old, and a big guy, with no other health complications. He is about a week ahead of you in his illness and had a similar progression: a flu that continued to get worse until he needed to go to the emergency room. Luckily, they transferred him to UNC hospital. They almost sent him to another place that didn't have ECMO. The good news was that he is doing really well. His lungs started to clear after four days on the machine. His parents assured me that the doctors here were the best and that you would start to get better soon.

There was so much happening that I was having trouble keeping track of it. I usually like to write things down to help me sort them out. (If I didn't have a number of "to do" lists in my pockets at any given time, I'm not sure I would know what to do next.) So I stopped by the gift shop to buy a spiral notebook where I could put things down. I decided to write it in the form of a journal addressed to Lil so that I could read it to her when she got better. I filled in from memory what had happened in the first few days.

When I came back to Lil's room early Tuesday morning, there was a new technician monitoring the two ECMO machines. He introduced himself as Gary, a ramrod straight, middle-aged guy with a down-home Southern accent. He was constantly in motion, going from one console to the other to make adjustments.

Lil's machine required more attention because she had only been on it a short time, so he spent most of the time on her side of the room. I asked him if he could explain to me what he was doing and he said, "Sure thing." But like a mother talking to her children while dinner is on the stove, he never stopped attending to his main task.

We stood between the ECMO machine and Lil's bed as he walked me through its operation. The machine was not very large, contained on a movable rack the size of a large computer cart. Multiple shelves hung off of it, loaded with electronic controls and monitors connected by a snake's nest of wires. But unlike a computer, the central portion of the machine had a core of blood-filled tubing going through it.

"The machine is just a big pump," Gary said. "Your blood goes in here (he pointed to the tube going into Lil's neck) and it comes out here (pointing to the line coming from her groin). This large circular thing is where the pumping is done. It's very gentle, so it doesn't damage the blood."

"Down here (he pointed with his flashlight to a red plastic cylinder) we have the oxygenator. That's where the blood exchanges gas with the atmosphere, just like in your lungs. On the side, coming from her body, it's dark red. But after it goes through the oxygenator, it gets much brighter." He held up the tube to show me. "This is the color we like to see."

He pointed to the console that he used to control the machine. "These monitors here let us keep track of what's going on in the blood. And these knobs let me control the flow from the machine into her body."

The levels of fluid in her body could be adjusted by adding more blood on the input side or taking liquid out on the other side. They had to add a lot of blood as her body got used to the machine, but eventually they would try to remove as much fluid as possible to allow her lungs to "dry out" and get rid of the secretions blocking them.

Then he made it clear where his domain ended, putting his fingers like scissors around the tubing midway between the machine and Lil's bed. "It's like there's an invisible line. I'm responsible for everything on the machine side of the circuit. But once the blood goes into her body, then the nurses are responsible."

Gary clearly loved these machines. Like a classic-car owner, he would pore over them, making sure there were no flaws. With the small flashlight he always kept in his pocket he would carefully inspect every inch of the clear plastic hoses, wiping them down with a soft cloth as he went. He was checking for clots in the tubing, a major potential complication.

One thing I was puzzled about was why the oxygen monitor on her finger read a lower value than the one on his console.

"That's a good question," he said. That phrase was the first thing he said to anything I asked.

"With the machine, I'm measuring the oxygen level in the blood directly after it flows past the oxygenator. That monitor (he pointed to the other side of Lil's bed) is connected to the sensor on her finger. It measures the oxygen after the blood has passed through her body. It's much lower, because her body has used up some of the oxygen we gave her. When her lungs are working again, then they'll add more oxygen to her blood and the level won't be so low. We'll know she's getting better when that number starts rising."

He pointed to the number on the screen. The oxygen saturation level measured by her finger monitor showed only 75 percent. For a normal person, it would be in the high 90s.

"Right now she's in a medically-induced coma and she doesn't need much oxygen. So that level is plenty. But we sure would like to see it go up. It's like with your kids—you can put a plate of food in front of them, but they won't eat it until they're ready."

We all loved talking to Gary and he loved to talk. At one moment he could be a very accomplished respiratory therapist and the next, a good ol' boy. It was so different from New England, where people keep to themselves. It was what Cate missed most about the South. We each had our favorite Gary-isms that we shared.

When we asked how he dealt with unexpected results, he replied: "Suppose you want a nice Chevelle, but instead you get the hardtop. That's still okay."

Had he been in the military? "No, sir. But my father was a retired drill sergeant, so that's just as good."

He told us what it was like when he came home late as a teenager:

"What time were you supposed to be home?"

"11 p.m., sir"

"What time did you arrive home?"

"11:30, sir"

"Is 11:30 before 11 p.m.?"

"No, sir."

When he was younger, he thought that he wanted to get away but as he got older, he realized he liked being a country boy, especially knowing that he had a choice and it wasn't forced on him. He had gotten himself a place in the country with some land now, and he was pretty happy.

Then he told me how he'd gotten into healthcare.

"I grew up not far from here. We were pretty poor, so we all had to work to help out. When I was in high school, I had a job at a gas station after school. And this man come around and said he would pay me three times as much if I came to work for him topping tobacco. Well, I swear, I have never done anything harder than that. And I said, 'God, if you can help me find a way to go to college, I will never ask you for anything else again.' Well, I got a scholarship to Duke, and I never have stopped being thankful for it."

Chapter 7

On the other side of the ECMO machine, Lil lay motionless. The stiff canula going into her neck ended with its tip only inches from her heart, so any movement could be dangerous.

She had been sedated since being put on the ventilator, but now she was also being given a paralytic agent to keep her muscles from moving at all. A large elastic bandage was wrapped around her head multiple times to secure the canula against her skull. The flexible hoses coming from the ECMO machine were anchored to the bed by strips of cloth clamped with forceps.

Ed, the pharmacist, came in early every morning to check on her and make sure the sedatives were working. She was a big challenge to him. Because she was young and small, it was hard to know the exact dose she needed. The walls of the ECMO tubing absorbed the drugs, so it was difficult to know how much of it was actually getting into her blood stream. And over time, she would develop a tolerance to anything he gave her, so he constantly had to be thinking of what to try next.

The paralytics were made from neurotoxins found in shellfish and there weren't that many options to try. He was often standing at the foot of her bed holding a clipboard when I arrived in the morning, like a head coach reviewing the game films and planning the strategy for next week.

The bed was surrounded by medical equipment. On her left side was the ECMO machine with its two large hoses carrying the blood back and forth. Also on that side was a rolling stand with pumps and IV lines that delivered antibiotics and fluids to her body. From under the sheets snaked a catheter that carried her urine into a plastic bag hanging below the bed rail.

Behind her left shoulder, a pump delivered a thin stream of beige liquefied food through a tube in her throat so her digestive system wouldn't shut down. Wires coming from multiple sensors on her body were bundled together at the top of the bed and fed to a rack of electronics behind her. Monitors there constantly updated readings for her temperature, heart rate, and blood oxygen, some in the form of numbers and others as luminous green lines traced out on the screens by a moving dot of light.

The ventilator sat in front of these monitors with a panel of knobs to control the pressure and a series of numbers reporting the volume of air in and out of her lungs. From the back of the machine came a hose that delivered the oxygenated air through a mouthpiece held by surgical tape over her face and then down into her lungs.

This didn't leave much room to maneuver around her. The nurses performed the intensive-care ballet as they weaved through the tangle of wires and tubes surrounding her, standing *en pointe* as they hung new bags of saline and leaping among the different monitors to silence the frequent alarms. When we wanted to be near Lil, the best spot was beside her left shoulder. Her head was turned slightly to the side, so we could talk into her left ear or stroke her hair. We could hold her hand as long as we were careful about the IV line in her forearm and the oxygen monitor attached to her index finger.

As we had been warned, her face was becoming extremely swollen in reaction to the ECMO machine. She had only recently lost all her baby fat over the summer and begun to look much more like a young woman than a kid.

Now, it was as though the clock was being reversed. Her beautiful face became pudgy with huge cheeks, as if she were holding her breath and pushing them out. Her neck developed rolls of skin like a severely overweight baby and the joints of her hands disappeared as the skin swelled up. She still looked feverish, and her skin was a deep, ruddy, purplish color that Cate couldn't stand to look at.

When Dr. Charles stopped in that afternoon, he assured us that this was normal and that the swelling would go down as she got used to the machine. At that point, they could start reducing the level of fluids. Hopefully we would see improvement in her lungs as the excess liquid was absorbed into her body.

Wednesday, 11/25 – Because of your size, Dr. Charles had to put a relatively small canula in your neck and groin. This restricted the blood flow in the tubing, so they couldn't get as much flow as they wanted and have to turn up the pressure to the highest level.

On Wednesday morning, they found that the oxygenator had a crack in it because of the high pressure they were using. Fortunately, your neighbor had come off the ECMO machine so his was now available to swap with yours. Unfortunately, this meant that you would have to go through the reaction to the machine again, so you would swell up again. They had to slow down and let you adjust to the machine and could not remove fluid from you as aggressively as they had. It was a pretty big setback, but it couldn't be avoided.

When we walked in on Wednesday morning, Dr. Charles was conferring with Gary and several other ECMO technicians in the middle of the room between Lil's bed and the other patient. I joined them and he filled me in on the growing cracks in the oxygenator and their plan to replace her machine. They could use the one that her neighbor had been on since he was no longer using it.

I glanced over and saw he was lying in his bed without even needing a respirator. They were weaning him off his sedation and he was acting like an angry drunk as he struggled to regain consciousness, shouting out incoherent phrases and fighting against the restraints that held him down.

The discussion seemed more like a bunch of guys talking about a plumbing job than medicine. The technicians described how they wanted to add a V-joint to the current tubing that would allow them to swap the new machine into the circuit. They discussed in detail where they would make the cut and where they would add the connectors and valve. The difficulty was that the machine had to be turned off briefly to do this and it was all that was keeping Lillian alive. So they wanted to make sure that there wouldn't be any mistakes when they did it. Dr. Charles okayed their plan and they left to practice it together.

Later in the morning, the team of infectious disease doctors came in to see Lil. They had taken many blood tests but none had come back positive, so they were still trying to determine the source of her illness. It was presumably H1N1, but she hadn't tested positive for it. Even so, they got special permission for her to go on a new experimental antiviral drug. She didn't fit the criterion for the clinical trials, but the company and the FDA allowed her to take it under a compassionate-use exemption.

These doctors were supposedly the elite of the medical hierarchy, solving problems that no one else could solve. But Lil's case had them stumped and their efforts seemed like comic relief relative to the ECMO team. Dr. Charles was a surgeon and his mission was to do the things that kept her alive RIGHT NOW, while theirs appeared to be coming up with unlikely scenarios for what could be causing it. He would listen politely to their latest theory or what tests they wanted to run, with a smile that said, "Go ahead," but indicated he wasn't waiting for them to figure it out.

That morning, the head of the team asked me to go to her dorm room and see whether I could find any potential sources of infection there. So, while the ECMO team was replacing the machine, Hannah and I went to Lil's room to search for possible causes of her illness.

The assistant dean of students met us at the entrance to the dorm and let us in. It was disconcerting to step into Lil's room, preserved in the shape she had left it when she went to the hospital. The bed was unmade and open books were still on her desk. I paused for a few minutes, remembering the last time I had seen the room when I came down for parents' weekend.

But Hannah wouldn't let me drift off and insisted that I get moving. We went through the motions of looking for anything suspicious, as if we were in an episode of "House," one of Lil's favorite shows. No dead animals, no drugs, which is what we suspected they wanted us to look for. Just a few moldy pears in the refrigerator and some unwashed dishes that we collected in a bag to bring back for testing.

We returned to Lil's hospital room in the afternoon. The change-over in the machine had gone well and she was stable. But the swelling, which in the morning had been a lot less than the day before, had now increased. Dr. Charles and Dr. Cairns stopped by to check on her progress and we were standing at the foot of her bed talking when the nurse from the reception desk came in. Two doctors from the university health services were there, she said, and wanted to talk to us.

I had no desire to meet with them. Lil had gone to the health services complaining of shortness of breath and they had just sent her back to her room with assurances that she would get better. They didn't do a blood test or give her a chest X-ray or prescribe Tamiflu. The assistant dean of students had probably called them because I'd told her how disgusted we were with the care Lil had received. There would be time to deal with this when Lil was better, but now was not the time.

Before I could answer that I didn't want to speak to them, Cate set her jaw and marched out of the room to where the two women were waiting beside the nurses' station.

They asked us about Lil's condition (though I'm sure they knew) and we gave them a brief update.

Then Cate started talking. "What are you doing for the students with H1N1?" she asked. "Lil's boyfriend Matt goes to Bowdoin and they set up a hall for students to go to when they start feeling sick. They stay there until their fever is gone."

One of the doctors said that they didn't have the staff for that, but Cate would have none of it.

"They make sure they are hydrated. They don't make them call their friends and beg them to bring over juice."

"We're a big state school," the same doctor answered. "We don't have those kinds of resources." But she didn't sound convinced herself.

"Don't you have libraries?" Cate said. "Don't you have gyms?"

They started to protest, but Cate was on a roll.

"Isn't there a rather large basketball arena that you could use?"

The women doctors were starting to back away from Cate, now.

"Do you realize that there is going to be another wave coming in the spring? The head of respiratory therapy told us she's terrified of what will happen if things got worse. There aren't enough respirators in the whole state of North Carolina. Tomorrow is Thanksgiving. How can you stay home and eat turkey knowing that you aren't prepared?"

By the time she was done, they were visibly shaken. They mumbled something and walked out. The nurses at the station were eyeing Cate with admiration, pumping their fist at her with a "You tell 'em" motion.

Cate watched the doctors leave the ICU then turned and walked back to Lil's room.

Chapter 8

Wednesday evening — Mark and Azi came over in the afternoon and brought the script of his play, "A New Dress for Mona", that you were cast in as the lead. That night, Hannah and I stood by your bed and read it out loud. I know that you would have been upset to hear us butchering it, but I wanted to hear it. I read Mona's part, and Hannah did most of the other characters. She especially liked being the mean guards as she tried to put on a tough voice. The play had a universal feel to it; I could tell because Hannah made the mother's voice sound Jewish (even though the characters were Iranian) and it still worked.

It told the true story of Mona, who was a young Bahá'í woman in Iran after the revolution. She and her father were imprisoned for their refusal to give up their faith. I could see how this character resonated so strongly with you. You are so similar in your temperament—outspoken, and willing to stand up for yourself and not back down. I cried at the part where she refused to leave her father even though he begged her to; it sounded just like you.

Hannah left after reading half the play and I read the remainder to myself standing by your bedside. The title refers to a dream that Mona has about getting a new dress. She is offered dresses of three different colors that symbolize different ways that you could live your life. At the end, Mona accepts the red dress for martyrdom and is executed for her beliefs. I stood by your bed for a long time with my eyes closed after I finished reading it, thinking about what this play must have meant to you.

I was amazed by Lillian's talent and interest in theater. I don't know where she got it, but there was nothing she liked better than acting.

Her attitude was different than mine when I was her age. To me, theater was all about Broadway shows and light operas. I grew up saturated with hearing the music from them. My father was a big do-it-yourselfer and my older brother and I spent most weekends indentured into working for him. Indentured as in "working for a fixed period of time in exchange for transportation, food, clothing, lodging and other necessities." We lived in a suburban neighborhood of houses that came in one of only two models and there was always something he wanted to do to make our house special: a fence in the backyard, a wet bar with a homemade refrigeration unit, air conditioners in each bedroom.

And with each project, we would have to listen to his music. It was the age of the hi-fi and my father had speakers wired into every room in the house so the music followed you everywhere you went.

"Seven Brides for Seven Brothers" was the score for remodeling the downstairs bathroom. "West Side Story" played when we paneled the recreation room. While the Jets and Sharks snapped their fingers, my brother and I swung sledgehammers and wielded crowbars to take down the old wall board.

In high school, I couldn't sing or dance but I hung out with friends who could. I would serve as an usher (within my talents) so that I could see repeat performances of my best friend, Larry, playing the cowboy Curly. During intermission, we ushers would sneak out to the tennis courts and drink beer so that by the finale we'd be standing in the aisles belting out "Oklahoma" with the rest of the chorus at the top of our lungs.

After I got older, my Broadway knowledge came in handy when it was the kids' bedtime. I would sing to them every night the songs that I knew by heart. I'd never thought I wanted to be a performer, but now I had an audience (albeit a captive one) and found myself looking forward to my nightly recitals. They would drift off to sleep as I crooned about the beautiful morning where the corn is as high as an elephant's eye.

Lillian started her own acting career in a two-week summer program where the kids wrote the play and then performed in it. I knew she'd had a good time but didn't realize how much it affected her until the following spring when we were watching the Oscar's. The four of us were curled up in our bed with a big bowl of popcorn.

Hannah was obsessed with fashion and fixated on the stars in their dresses. She had to comment on every one as they strode down the red carpet.

Lil, as usual, kept her own counsel and spoke much less. But when Catherine Zeta-Jones strode up to the stage to accept her best supporting actress award, Lil turned to Cate and said, "That's going to be me some day."

Lots of kids could make comments like that, but Lillian didn't say things lightly. She had great determination when she set her mind to something. Just a few years before, after coming home from a Passover Seder, she had used a similar voice to announce that next year, she would read the four questions in Hebrew. Before you could say "Mazel Tov," we had joined a temple and three years later, Hannah and Lil had a joint Bat Mitzvah. So, when Lil said she was going to be an actress it was something to be considered.

The following summer, after finishing eighth grade, she was in a production of the musical "Oliver" and played one of the chorus of urchins that takes in the main character. She also had a solo as a milkmaid walking the streets of London, singing a simple song asking, "Any milk today?" in a hauntingly beautiful voice.

Off to a good start by my reckoning, her life as a song-and-dance woman came to an abrupt end after the next show she was in, a production by the high-school drama program. Cast as a sailor in a nautical chorus, she disappeared over the side of the ship before the end of the first act, never to be seen again.

She didn't want to hear any speeches from me about paying her dues or waiting for her turn. She didn't like the whole ethos of the high-school program, where there were only a few highly competitive parts and the rest were backups. Plus, there was only one show a year. So she found an alternative.

Instead of high-school theatrics, she focused on the community theater program. This group was organized around a series of drama fests that were held three times a year. Over the course of two days, they would put on a series of one-act plays that were acted in and also directed by kids from the middle school and high school. The older kids worked with the younger kids, teaching them what they knew.

Most importantly, each participant was in at least two of the plays, and had a lot of chances to participate. There was also one main production directed by the head of the program for which judges from the theater world gave critiques at the end of each show, explaining what they liked about each piece and what could be better. The rehearsal schedule was intense, with only 10 weeks between the auditions and the festival performance. But because it was held multiple times a year, Lil could get a lot more experience.

I hand-held a video camera to record each of her roles and through the years, it was like a flip book watching her get more mature with each festival. One-act plays are not something that are produced commercially, so the material was often surprising. In one Christopher Durang script, Lil played a mother who was supposed to be both beautiful and a bitch—she sent her daughter away to an orphanage and only reappeared to receive her dying father's money. Although Lil was only 15 years old, it was scary how convincing she was.

She developed a special talent for playing earnest young woman, able to deliver her lines with an utterly convincing sincerity that came from her own beautiful soul. In real life, she could be cynical and sharp, with a wit that cut to the core of a situation. It often got her in trouble with friends who couldn't understand her.

But she also had a core of honesty that stemmed from a belief that things ought to be fair. This came out when she was in "The Brick and The Rose," a play about a teen-age boy who becomes a drug addict. Her character begs him to stop, asking him what has happened to the person she knew. The words could easily sound trite, but she delivered them with such honest feeling. I looked around and saw teen-age boys openly crying in empathy with her character's pain. Teen-age boys and open displays of emotion aren't two things that I normally associate with each other.

One spring, they even put on a production of "Grease" and I got to satisfy my Broadway cravings when Lil played Sandy, the female lead. Luckily for the people sitting next to me, I was holding the video camera, so I couldn't sing along. Listening to her sing "Hopelessly Devoted" was one of the high points of my life.

In the final scene, she came on the stage in a tight, sexy costume, a shocking transformation from the goody-two-shoes character she started out as. The gasps of surprise from the audience confirmed what a beautiful young woman she was. Later, our friend David told Matt that he had better forget what he had seen on the stage.

But to Lil, this wasn't really acting. She hated the falseness, the big expressions and the obvious setups. She put me in my place when I praised the performance of one of the other actresses who she thought was over-the-top: "I like it best when it doesn't seem like acting."

In her senior year, she directed a play for the first time. She chose to make an adaptation of "Of Mice and Men," shortening it to fit within the one-hour,one-act time frame. It tells the story of two brothers, George and Lenny, looking for work as depression-era farmhands. Lenny, physically strong, is mentally handicapped, and George is struggling to help them get by.

She decided to take a chance on an inexperienced 13-year-old girl named Erika, for the lead of George. It was a risk, but she felt it was worthwhile. At least until her lead actress started letting her down.

"I don't know how to make her more committed to the role, to really care about it," she told me after I picked her up from one rehearsal. I could hear the frustration in her voice and sense the rising fear that the production wasn't going to work.

"She's only 13," I said.

"So what? I was 13, too. If you say you're going to do something, you do it."

She called Erika every night, trying to invoke in her the same passion that she had for acting. One afternoon, she had her George and Lenny come over our house to work without the rest of the cast. Lil's latest theory was that maybe the girl was too young to really understand the part. The boy who played George was older and more experienced, so Lil had asked him to come, too.

While I was in the kitchen preparing dinner, they worked in the living room so I overheard what they were doing. Lil gave them exercises to try, imagining different feelings, anything to get them to loosen up and express themselves, but to do it honestly. While I was chopping vegetables, I could hear the sounds of grunts, squeals of laughter and stomping of feet. I stopped what I was doing and went over to look through the door when I heard Lil screaming at her.

What I saw was Lil holding her hand to Erika's belly, explaining how to vocalize what she was feeling. Was Lil really yelling at her, letting out her own frustration, or was she being a good teacher?

Erika seemed unperturbed so I went back to the kitchen wondering if anyone could even tell where the line was between real-life and acting?

At the same time as she was directing, Lil had the lead in the main production of "12 Angry Jurors" (modified from "12 Angry Men" to suit the half-female cast). The last few weeks of rehearsal were difficult, working on the two plays simultaneously. We could tell she was exhausting herself with rehearsals four nights a week on top of her usual load of schoolwork, but it was what she loved most and she wouldn't cut back.

Both plays were performed on the same day of the drama festival in the high- school auditorium. "Of Mice and Men" was on first at 3 in the afternoon. It had its flaws—the physically imposing Lenny was only 5-foot-4 and the tough-as-nails George was a 13-year-old girl—but it went off surprisingly well. Simple-minded Lenny accidentally kills the wife of the boss and he meets up with George by the banks of the river where they had been camping. George tells Lenny to imagine the rabbit farm they always dreamed of having together and, as the search dogs are coming closer, shoots him to save him from being captured. Erika nailed the final speech, delivering it in a way that felt believable and sincere.

Lil came out with the actors for their applause. The judges gave her and the cast some good suggestions and she seemed content with how it had gone. But she didn't have time to think about it. She had to get ready for her acting part.

When "12 Angry Jurors" went on at 8 p.m., she played the same part that Henry Fonda played in the movie, the one who convinces all the other jurors to change their votes. The cast was costumed in '50s-style clothes, guys in suits and tie, the women in dresses and skirts. The set was a simple jury room with a long table.

Lil's performance was so perfect for her, articulate and passionate, yet still believable, the one person who would speak up for the sake of justice.

The judges gave her an award for best actress. It was one of her last productions during high school, and it was a great way to finish.

After the play, we stood in the corridor leading to the classrooms that served as the dressing rooms as the young actors and actresses filed out into the arms of adoring fans and parents. Cate and I got big hugs when she saw us and we gave her the flowers we had brought for her.

Then we stepped back to let her be surrounded by her friends and the rest of the cast. I watched all the different kinds of smiles that played across her lively face as she greeted different people. It made me realize what the word "radiant" meant. She was lit up from within.

As I was enjoying the vicarious pleasure of seeing Lil reap the rewards of doing something she loved and worked hard at, a finger touched my shoulder and an attractive woman leaned over to talk to me. I didn't know her, but through the noise she was able to explain that she was Erika's mother. She wanted me to know how wonderful she thought Lil was for giving her daughter a chance and working with her so closely.

I smiled as I thought fleetingly of the screaming session I'd witnessed, then thanked her. In the Broadway version, this is when the music would come up reprising the actress's theme song before the curtain fell. The sound I heard was the squeals of the teen-age cast members telling each other how great they had done. It was just as good.

Chapter 9

Thursday, 11/26 — Around 2 a.m., the nurses from the ICU called our room and told us to come to the hospital immediately. Dr. Charles had warned us that he would be honest with us about your condition so we knew it must be serious. We fumbled into our clothes and drove over to the hospital. Hannah dropped us off at the front entrance and went to park the car in the garage.

Cate and I burst past the guard at the front entrance, yelling that we had to hurry to the ICU and waving my hospital ID as we went by. He knew who we were and didn't make us stop.

We ran through the empty corridors of the hospital, covering the long distance as fast as we could, running too hard to talk. My mind raced as fast as my feet. I was hoping that it would be something they could control, but I couldn't imagine what that could be. If it weren't serious, they wouldn't have called us.

When we got to the ICU, we had to put on gowns and masks before we could go to Lillian's bed. The first few times we did this, I thought they were concerned about us infecting Lil while she was on the ECMO but it was the opposite. They were still concerned that she was infectious and didn't want anyone else exposed.

Dr. Charles walked in while we were still getting into the protective gear. He had just arrived. When the nurse had called him because there was some bleeding in Lil's breathing tube, he instructed the nurse to call us also. He was going to look into her lungs and survey the extent of the bleeding.

"This could be a game-changer," he said as he pulled on his surgical scrubs. "We've had to make her blood very thin to keep clots from forming."

We didn't say anything, only nodded, trying to show that we understood.

The nurse told him that everything was ready and he stepped up to the left side of Lil's bed, where the nurse had laid out the instruments.

We squeezed in front of the ECMO machine about six feet behind him, craning to see what he was doing.

He turned the TV monitor toward us so that we could see the same image he did. Hannah arrived and stood beside us as he inserted the fiber-optic camera into Lil's breathing tube and threaded it down through her airway.

As the camera worked its way down, we could see the inside of Lillian's lungs. The walls of her airway were pinkish white, with rings of cartilage giving it a ribbed appearance. The passageways started out wide and got thinner as the camera went deeper. Like following the inside of a cave, he kept inserting the probe into smaller and smaller pathways until he couldn't proceed any further.

He hadn't wanted to use the scope before because the probe itself can cause bleeding, but now he had to see for himself what was happening. Although there was some blood in the secretions, it wasn't the hemorrhaging he had feared. Other regions looked similar: pink tissue with a few small streaks of red on the walls of her lungs. When he was finished, he withdrew the scope and a radiology technician came in to take an X-ray.

Dr. Charles took off his gloves and turned to the nurse who had been caring for her that evening. "Why did you call me?" he asked in a measured tone, trying to keep his voice neutral.

"There was some blood in the tube. You told me to call if there were any problems," he answered.

Dr. Charles sighed, the way you do when your child does something that's not what you wanted, but is technically what you told them. The nurse was a young man and like a lot of the staff, he was still inexperienced in working with ECMO patients.

Dr. Charles picked up the tubing that went to the respirator and looked at it, then turned to us and explained that the blood was likely just due to irritation from the tube in her throat but wasn't serious. He confirmed that the lung tissue looked pretty good, just what I thought I had seen.

Then why weren't her lungs working? Because the problem wasn't in the passageways we could see. It was at the smallest levels, where the air exchanges with the blood. That was the part that was clogged with secretions.

Cate, Hannah and I were in a state of shock. We had all been fearing the worst, and now, suddenly, there was nothing new. Maybe Dr. Charles was used to this, but we weren't. Our adrenaline had pumped us up to a state of emergency and now we were left hanging.

Dr. Charles pulled up the X-ray on the computer system and he called us over to look at it. Amazingly, we could see the tube snaking down from her neck with the tip on its end stopping near her heart. It was all so real, yet so impossible to believe. This was actually the inside of our daughter's body.

"This looks like it's shifted," he said, pointing out how the tube was farther in than he wanted it to be. Moving it required a surgical procedure and he asked us to step outside while he repositioned it. When he was done, he came out to the nurses' station to talk to us.

"That helped," he said. "Her oxygen levels went up after I was done"

We all walked out of the ICU in a daze, Dr. Charles coming with us. It was about 4 in the morning. I told him I was sorry that he had had to come in and he laughed. He was more worried about us, especially Cate, who was looking pale and shaky. There was a room for the doctors to take naps in and he wanted her to have his key to it. She could use it anytime she needed to get some rest, he said. She protested but he insisted, and they left so he could show Cate where it was.

Hannah and I looked at each other, still in disbelief. "What do you want to do now?" I asked her. It was too late to go back to the Ronald Macdonald house, so we decided to go into the lobby and try to get some sleep.

The lobby was a big, round corridor that wrapped around the front of the building, connecting several different hospitals together. It was designed as a space for people to meet and mingle, and there were many clusters of large comfortable chairs where people could sit and wait. Huge windows rose from the ground to the second story. This gave it an open, sunlit feeling during the day, but when we arrived it was still dark.

Hannah pulled two chairs up next to each other, spread out across them, and soon fell asleep. I pulled up a coffee table to put my legs on, but only dozed briefly.

As the sun rose, the lobby grew increasingly busier. I was so exhausted, I simply lay there and watched the panorama of people marching by. I felt like I was looking at the giant aquarium in Boston that we had taken the kids to see. The fish swam around the tank but didn't mix, each species keeping to its own level.

The hospital had its own variety of species. There were schools of happy families carrying vases of flowers with pastel ribbons, coming to see the new baby. A pod of older relatives followed closely behind a young boy as he proudly led them, pushing his grandmother in a wheelchair. There were solitary people darting by, walking deliberately, rushing to the elevator and not looking around as they walked.

Then there were those more like us, the ones who stayed on the deeper levels. We saw them in the cafeteria at all hours, talking quietly to each other or hanging their heads over a cup of coffee. One family's mother had had a stroke and she probably wasn't going to survive. A young woman had a child who had been burned severely and had been in the hospital for months. We might see them at any hour, and we would sometimes nod to each other in recognition.

Hannah slept until around 9 and then we went back to Lil's room. I went up to the bed and held her hand for a while. I always liked to talk to her when I came into the room, letting her know we were there and telling her what was new. I recounted the story of how we had come in the middle of the night, but everything had been okay and so we had gone to take a nap in the lobby. I told her that she would love Dr. Charles, and how I couldn't wait until she was better so that she could meet him.

About 45 minutes later, Cate came back. She had slept for a few hours and looked a lot better. It was a strange sense of relief that we all felt. Our worst fears hadn't been realized, and the numbers on the machines were looking a little better than the day before, since Dr. Charles had adjusted the tubing.

But things still weren't improving enough.

"Can you believe it's Thanksgiving?" Hannah said. Lillian's favorite holiday. Just the day before, Hannah had joked that Lil was bound to get better today. "Wouldn't it be like her to get better on Thanksgiving? Just like a movie!"

I reached up and turned on the television to the Macy's parade. Since the time when the kids were babies, it had been a Thanksgiving routine for Cate to turn on the parade and march along to the bands and imitate the dancers on the floats. "Come on, Lil," Cate called as she pumped her legs up and down and danced around the room.

The nurses looked at us like we were crazy, but we didn't care.

Gary, the ECMO technician, came in to say goodbye before he left for his Thanksgiving break. He had just finished a shift in a different ICU.

"I have a 21-year-old daughter. I can't imagine anything worse than what you're going through," he said and gave me a bear hug. "We're going to do the very best we can for her."

We had gotten many invitations for Thanksgiving dinner but none of us wanted to socialize. It would have been impossible to be around other people today, trying to talk about anything but this. It was painful enough thinking about our past holidays. In any other year, I'd have gotten up at 6 to get the turkey in the oven and then we'd have gone out for breakfast. And Lil had been so excited about coming home for the first time since college had started. We ought to have been sitting down to eat right about now.

"Well, I'm hungry," Hannah said. "Let's go to the K&W."

The K&W was a cafeteria and it seemed as good as anything else. It was packed when we arrived. We got our trays and filled them up with plates of turkey with stuffing and yams with marshmallows, then added mashed potatoes and collard greens and glasses of sweet iced tea. We carried them to a table and ate as best we could. As horrible as things were, I was glad that Hannah was with us.

Afterward, we returned to the hospital and settled back in. There were several chairs in Lil's room where we could sit without being in the nurses' way. We would alternate between reading or standing by Lil's bed, stroking her arm and talking to her. I would sit and watch the numbers on the monitors, hoping to see them start to rise. We weren't allowed to use our cell phones in the ICU, so we would take breaks and go into a corridor nearby where the reception was adequate. Cate had many people calling her wanting to know how we were and she spent a lot of time out there.

At around 5 p.m., we were surprised to see Dr. Charles again. He was standing at the edge of the curtain surrounding Lil's room.

"Don't you ever sleep?" I asked him.

He put back his head and laughed. "Lillian's my girl. I have to check up on her."

He stood aside so that we could see the woman standing behind him. "I'd like you to meet my wife."

"I'm very pleased to meet you," she said after Dr. Charles introduced us. She was a beautiful woman, with a lovely Nigerian accent.

Dr. Charles explained that he wanted her to see what he did. Now, he said, she could understand why he had to leave at a moment's notice.

They had already had their Thanksgiving dinner and his mother-in-law was watching their two kids. While he was talking to us, she kept her eyes on Lillian the entire time. Her eyes were filled with such tenderness, the kind a mother shows.

"So young. So beautiful" she said. She turned to Dr. Charles, "You have to do everything you can for her."

"I am," he said. "Believe me, I am."

Chapter 10

When Lillian was younger, she played softball in little league. As the pitcher, she never minded being in tight situations. She might not always win, but she wanted to be the one with the ball.

She was on the smallish side for her age, but she had good form and she knew how to put all of her body into her pitching. When she stood on the pitcher's mound, she was as frightening in her intensity as a 10-year-old girl could be.

Off the mound, she was a big-hearted, smiling, ponytailed bundle of joy, but when she was pitching, she was focused on only one thing. Not in a mean way, but her eyes were like lasers and she was clearly in another world, one that existed only for her and the batter.

She had her routine down. First, she would stare at the batter, then look down at the big ball in her glove as she started her windup. Her arm would windmill all the way around while she took a big step toward the plate, letting go of the ball just as it passed her hip, with her signature little twist-of-the-wrist for added spin. When she was on, the ball would be rising as it crossed the plate and the batter would have barely started to move the bat when the umpire called a strike.

It wasn't always like that, and she gave up her share of walks. But in this league, it was an achievement to make three outs before allowing the maximum of six runs in an inning and she was about as reliable as they came. Plus, she really loved being in the middle of the action.

A lot of the other girls, well, you could say their minds were somewhere else. When a ball was hit hard, it wasn't unusual to have to yell to get the outfielder's attention because she was busy picking dandelions.

Lil was pretty excited when her coach called to tell us she was invited to a pitching clinic. The league offered it every year, given by a woman who was a semi-pro pitcher and also gave lessons at her softball school, if we were interested. It was by invitation only and would be held at the high school on Saturday morning.

We were the first ones out at the field that morning, waiting for everyone else to show up. Lil and I had both brought our gloves as we'd been instructed.

At about 9 a.m., the instructor drove up in a large, gun-metal-grey pick-up. She reached into the back and pulled out a large, white plastic bucket filled with softballs. She nodded a cursory hello in our direction and then headed off to the pitcher's mound with the balls.

She walked around the mound, inspecting it, and doing squats and other stretches while we waited for the other girls and their parents to show up. We were soon a group of about a dozen, congregating around the edge of the backstop.

She walked back from the mound, looking at the ground. When she reached the group, she looked up, making it clear she was ready to get started.

It was then I realized what a remarkably large woman she was. She must have been 6-foot-2, with some seriously strong muscles. She was wearing a snug-fitting shirt and stretch baseball pants and had short, blonde hair that stuck out under a red cap. The look in her eyes was frighteningly reminiscent of the one I saw in Lillian's when she pitched.

I looked over at Lil, who had a huge smile of excitement, like she had finally found her tribe and was about to be inducted.

The woman told us her name was Sheila and asked who wanted to be a pitcher. Six T-shirted arms shot up immediately.

Then she told us about her background, naming some teams she had been on that were clearly important in the world of women's semi-pro softball. What she wanted to impress most on the girls was that good pitching came from the legs, which on her were truly impressive.

Then she picked up her glove off the ground and went to the mound. "It's important that you follow through with your hips. That's where all the power comes from," she explained as she wound up and threw a pitch.

It came out of her hand like a rocket and slammed into the chain link fence behind the plate.

"How fast was that?" one of the other fathers asked.

"Oh, probably about 80," she responded.

She gave a few more pointers, following each one by a chest-high strike that rocked the backstop.

The girls looked like they were in a trance.

"Who here can catch for me?" she asked.

All of the girls raised their hands, but she waved them off and said, "I mean the parents."

I looked at the other adults. None of them had gloves or showed any inclination to volunteer.

"My daddy can," Lil piped up cheerfully.

With a sinking feeling, I looked down at the glove in my hand and then I heard the word "Okay" come out of my mouth.

I walked over to the plate, balancing in my mind the relative cost of appearing like a coward in front of my daughter versus a broken face. I could feel two pathways in my life diverging and I, unable to choose the rational one, went into a crouch behind the plate.

My mitt felt extremely small as I held it in front of my face while she went into her windup. My muscles were in self-defense mode and started pushing my glove forward even before she released the ball.

When it came out of her hand, it didn't just come straight at me but hopped around, dancing on the air. The mitt felt weightless as I tried to keep it in front of the ball, which was going faster than my brain could react. I'm not sure you could say I caught it as much as that she hit my glove perfectly.

I threw it back and we did it again. The next one moved around a little more, but I managed to keep the glove in front of it and caught it in the edge of the webbing.

She looked over at Lillian.

"Those were only about half-speed," she said. "Should I throw it full speed?"

She went into her windup and I heard a scream come from behind me.

"STOP!" Lillian shouted. "Don't hurt him."

The pitcher stopped and laughed. "Most kids say, 'Go ahead and throw it as hard as you can'."

Lillian ran around and threw her arms around my neck. The emperor's thumb had turned up. The lion wouldn't get to eat the slave today.

Sheila lined up the girls along the fence and put them through some drills, working on snapping their hips forward as they finished their pitching motion. It didn't look quite the same on them as it did on Sheila, like watching them trying to do dances that were meant for older girls. They each got to throw her a few pitches and then she wrapped it up, letting us know how to reach her if we wanted more private instruction.

We went home and had lunch, and that afternoon Lil asked if I would catch some for her.

I got out our bucket of balls from the garage and we went to our usual spot on the lawn, alongside the garden where the slope was pretty level. We didn't talk much as she practiced her delivery, but it was clear that she was trying to translate the mechanics that Sheila had taught her into her own version. Eventually it became part of her style. She would pull her trailing leg up quickly until it hit her planted front leg, and she would finish her delivery by standing on one foot like a bowler after letting go of the ball. She developed a permanent black-and-blue mark on the back of her left calf where her right foot slammed into it.

When we were done, as we walked back to the house, I asked her whether she wanted me to call Sheila about getting some more lessons.

"No," she said, "I'm good."

She had a few more good seasons of pitching for little league. At the tryouts for her last summer of eligibility, she had trouble catching pop-ups, even though she was always a good fielder. We attributed it to the lights in the gym. She pitched for the ninth-grade high-school girls' team, but it wasn't as much fun anymore. She'd started to be afraid that she was going to get hit by the ball. We thought that it was because the hitters were getting better and she couldn't overpower them the way she once had. Because she wasn't very big, a lot of her talent came from having great form and making the best of what she had. We thought that the size of the other kids was starting to make up for that.

After we found out about her eyesight, we realized that was the reason. She couldn't see the ball when it came off the bat until it was close to her, so she had even less time to react than a normal pitcher would. Only her great reaction time had kept her playing as long as she did.

Chapter 11

Friday, 11/28 – The oxygenator cracked again because of the high pressure they needed to use. This time, instead of replacing the entire machine, they just replaced the oxygenator so your allergic response would be less. They also added a "y" joint so that they could put in a second oxygenator, which would make it easier to get higher flow without increasing the pressure. We learned that they were doing the same thing in Michigan where Dr. Charles had trained.

We had several visitors during the day and we sat with them in the lobby since there were too many for the NSICU. The doctor from pediatrics came by, very excited because she was going to escort the basketball team to the children's burn unit. I ran back to the NSICU and got your script from the play for them to sign. The team came in around 4 p.m. and it was amazing to see how young they were. Although they were very tall, they weren't really much older than you.

They posed to let us take pictures with our cell phones and were sweet about all signing your script. They seemed to be really affected when they heard about you being sick, since you are one of their classmates.

Last year at this time, our biggest concern was Lillian getting her college applications done. It's unfortunate how stressful that has become, especially in the Northeast.

Look at Lil and her friends. Smart young women from a good high school. Great grades, lots of outside interests. Delightful, clever, funny. Kids who are so special, and they're made to feel so run-of-the-mill. Even perfect grades weren't enough to guarantee admission to a place like Brown. Maybe we would have done better to stay in Albuquerque, where Lil would have stood out more, instead of being treated like part of a herd.

Lil wanted to apply to the University of North Carolina at Chapel Hill for early decision, so she had to have her application in early. Cate and I were concerned that she not wait until the last minute. Lil could be a procrastinator.

But she wouldn't talk to us about it. Every time I tried to bring it up, she threw her hands up and stormed out or ran into her room.

I finally made her sit down at the end of October to talk to me. It was a Friday afternoon when just the two of us were home. I assumed the problem was the essay. Most kids can't face it and will do anything to avoid it. So I asked her when she was going to start.

She furrowed her brow and told me that she had already written the essay. The problem was she couldn't fill out the application online because the type was too small. The computer program she had to expand text didn't work on the forms.

"Why didn't you ask me to help?"

"You told me I had to do it myself," she replied.

I guess I had said that. But I hadn't meant filling out the forms. I meant she needed to write the essays herself.

I told her not to worry. Then I called our friend Thom, and his partner Kevin, to come over for brunch on Saturday. "Could you bring your laptops with you?" I asked. "Lil needs help filling out her applications."

We set up everybody's computer on the kitchen table the next morning. Cate was at work, since she saw her acupuncture patients on Saturday. Kevin worked on the common application, entering Lil's address, birthdate, etc. Thom worked on the list of extracurriculars that she had put together, making it fit into the proper format.

I asked Lil to give me the essay she had written so I could enter it into the website.

Thom said "Oh, read it to us," and Lil did:

When my English teacher introduced Plato's Allegory of the Cave as: "The most important story EVER!" a few kids rolled their eyes, but as he enthusiastically danced around the room I began to understand what he meant by "most important." Plato's allegory is about a man who, after seeing nothing of the world but shadows on a cave's wall, bravely journeys through his cave to finally see sunlight. Metaphorically, the allegory can be applied to every person as they travel from ignorance to truth, whether it be emotional, social, intellectual, or any other aspect of life. "Many people will never truly see the sun," Mr. Scott continued. "They will keep it real with the shadows being that they are too ignorant or careless to search for enlightenment." I will admit that, like all high-schoolers, I still have years of education before I can see the proverbial sun of knowledge. However, with respect to another part of my life, I have seen the sun.

Sophomore year of high school I was diagnosed with a degenerative eye disease known as Stargardt's. Most people will never experience the function-loss of a sense, something that is so engrained in our every movement that we are barely conscious of its existence. It's hard to imagine a world without music, Lewis Black (shout out to UNC grad!), or chocolate chip cookies, but luckily I've still got those. I may not be able to play softball anymore, but it's opened the door to rowing crew for me. I may have to spend longer on my homework, but I'm proud that even though I can't read the newspaper I am still a member of NHS and the only kid in my British Literature class to receive honors. I don't think a disability makes someone a better person, but I feel that after conquering such an obstacle I've proven I refuse to be held back.

I don't let my eyesight define me, but I recognize that it is a part of me. It doesn't stop me, but I know I have limits. I value and maintain my independence, but after not being able to get my license or see the letters on the board, I've had to allow myself to depend on a supportive community much more than if I were fully sighted. As my eyesight degenerates, I know I will have to continue to rely on my community, wherever that may be. After I traveled the campus at UNC Chapel Hill, I knew I'd found a community that would embrace my differences; one that would see me as a person first and visually impaired second. I'm not looking for pity from my community; I want people to understand that I harbor no feelings of remorse or regret for my genetic composition. In many ways, my lack of sight has opened my eyes. I appreciate the things I can still see, and I feel confident in saying that I have taught my community to appreciate the things they can see a little more as well. If I am admitted to UNC Chapel Hill, I know I will add to your community the wisdom and experience that comes with loss. I have seen one proverbial sun; I want to be one of the many students who will be guided by UNC to see countless others.

While she read, I looked away from the others, not wanting to make eye contact, afraid if I did I would start crying.

I wasn't alone. Thom stared up at the ceiling, Kevin out the windows at the bare garden.

"That's good," I managed to squeeze out when she was done.

"Yeah," she said. "Some of my friends say they're jealous that I have my eyesight to talk about."

She said it so matter-of-factly, with no trace of irony in her voice. No bitterness. I often wondered how I would have reacted if I were in Lil's shoes. Would I have hated everything and everyone?

Not Lil. Her failing eyesight was just a part of herself that she had to accept. Her teacher of the visually impaired told me she asked Lil how she felt about it. "It is what it is," Lil had replied.

Don't you start crying or I'll cry too, she'd say to me. She needed for me to be strong and help her, not to feel sorry for her. She wouldn't share her fears with me, the worries I know she had. Sometimes I heard her crying in her room but I wouldn't ask her to talk about it. I was afraid there was nothing I could say, angry that there was nothing I could do.

Instead, I told her that I would always be there if she needed me, and tried to show her whenever I could. She didn't want to have to ask her friends for rides all the time so I never complained if she called me at the last minute (I know that I am very lucky to have the flexibility to work from home when I need to). I would sit in the line of cars at school to pick her up, watching for her. I'd get out of the car and try to wave discreetly so that she could see me. She'd smile with relief when she figured out where I was and then come skipping over to me. Sometimes we'd stop for a snack, but usually I took her straight to the house where she baby-sat for two children in the neighborhood, Sam and Sophia. She'd stay with them for the rest of the afternoon until their parents got home from work.

Lil finished her application to UNC in time to be considered for early decision. Students don't wait for the fat envelope to arrive in the mail anymore to find out whether they've gotten in. As soon as she got home from school on January 15, she went on the computer to learn she had been accepted.

This was very exciting. Not many people from Rhode Island get accepted to UNC each year. She was very proud of herself, and it took a lot of pressure off of her. Her friends still had to wait months to find out where they would go to college.

The early decision wasn't binding, so she was still free to look at other schools. Her choice got more complicated when she was accepted to Brown in April. Lil had been interviewed by one of the trustees, who was really impressed by her and wanted her to come.

She called Lil and made a strong case for why it was such a great school. We took a tour of the campus (which she hadn't done before, even though she had been to my office many times) and met with the director of the disabilities services. She showed Lil a room and discussed with her what they could do and where she could live in order to have good access.

It was a difficult decision, but not because one was where her mother went to school and the other was where her father taught. We truly wanted to do what was best for Lil. The disabilities services were great in both places. It was clear that in either case, she would get the things she needed to help her succeed (like digitizing her books, getting notes, extra time for exams, etc.).

The intangibles were more difficult to judge. If she stayed in Providence, we would always be able to help her. Thom taught at the graduate program in drama at Trinity Rep and could also help. Lil knew her way around and wouldn't have trouble getting oriented. The children of my colleagues who went there said it was a different world and they didn't feel like they were still at home.

On other hand, UNC was sunny and Southern. Cate often talked about what a wonderful place it was when she went there. She liked to say that Jesse Helms called it little Russia because it was so liberal. But most importantly, it was away from home. Not in Providence, just 10 miles from where she had grown up.

We told her it was up to her. We would be okay either way. Both were great schools.

As the deadline approached, Lil had a hard time deciding. She kept going back and forth, and we listened patiently as she talked about the pros and cons of each place. I really couldn't guess which way she would go.

On the final day before the decisions were due, she told us she was choosing UNC. Although it was scary, this was her greatest chance to be independent. When she was older and her eyesight was worse, she might want to live near us so we could help her. But now, while she still could, she wanted to go out on her own.

Chapter 12

Saturday, 11/28 —The doctors were originally hoping to see some improvement by today but there hasn't been any. Your lungs are still very stiff.

I asked Dr. Charles about the possibility of a lung transplant if things don't improve. He was going to talk to the transplant team about it. They may not allow it because they aren't sure why you got sick. Or they may because the disease is confined to your lungs. I pray that we don't have to consider it.

They had put Lil back on a conventional ventilator after they put her on the ECMO machine. This type of ventilator pushes air into the lungs at a set pressure for a certain amount of time. It also allowed the doctors and staff to measure the increase in volume with pressure, called the tidal volume. When it blew into Lil's lungs, the volume was only on the order of 80 to 100 mL (mL stands for milliliters), less than half a cup. Like trying to blow up a balloon made of very stiff elastic. When they started, the volume was only 30 mL, so this was some improvement. But for normal lungs, the number should be around 500 mL.

We had hoped to see more improvement by this point. The H1N1 patient in the bed next to hers had already been discharged after only four days on ECMO.

But Dr. Charles told us not to be discouraged. According to a recent paper, patients in Australia remained on it for 7 to 10 days.

The initial virus was probably no longer there, he told us. What she was fighting now was her own body's massive overreaction to the initial viral attack. It often turns off just like a switch. When the body realizes that the immune response is no longer needed, it reabsorbs the secretions and the lungs can start to work again.

But right now, her lungs were still filled with fluid in the smallest recesses, where the gases exchange across the cell membrane and get into the blood system. This is why her lungs appeared completely white in the X-rays. They were as dense as her liver, when they should be like tissue paper.

"Massive overreaction." I used that term later when I stood by Lil's bed and talked to her. I often had conversations with her, to tell her about what was going on, or to report what the doctors had said, even though she couldn't respond or understand.

"You know how you always overreact when Hannah makes you mad?" I asked her. "Just let it go. Just let it go."

Whenever we had free time, we looked at the "Prayers for Lillian" Facebook page. Hannah and Lil had signed me up for Facebook two summers earlier, while we were at the beach on vacation, but after we got back, they both unfriended me (pretty demoralizing), so I had never used it.

At first, I thought the page would mostly be useful to let us keep people updated about her status. But it soon turned into a community of people offering support and prayers. Her UNC friends put up recent photos that we hadn't seen before, like little bursts of sunshine in the gloom. Had she always been so beautiful and I just wasn't aware of it? Or had she become more radiant since leaving home?

We could see the comments appear from different communities as the news of her illness spread. They came from so many people that it was overwhelming. On just this one day, there were more than 100, from all phases of her life and ours—high school and college, from Rhode Island, North Carolina and all over the world.

Lillian I can't tell you how many times I've gone to pick up my phone and call you to tell you about something I thought you'd find hilarious or to just ask your opinion or just to talk because I was bored and I'm waiting anxiously for the day when i get to talk to you again. I'm thinking of you constantly and sending you all the love and positive energy in the world. Please get better soon, Lil. I love you so much and I just want to see you and your gorgeous smile as soon as possible.

November 29, 2009 at 10:56pm ·

In the early morning there were posts from people who checked the website as soon as they woke up. In the evening there was another burst as people checked up on her at the end of the day and wished her well for the night:

Good night Lil, sweet dreams! Tomorrow is going to be a good day, i can just feel it! I love you and cant stop thinking about you ♥

November 30, 2009 at 12:47am

All day long, people would write to share kind words and urge her to keep fighting. Rowers from the boat club said pull harder, like when you're racing. Church groups wrote that they were putting her in their prayers. Pictures and links to her favorite songs were posted with descriptions of listening to them with her. Someone even went over to our house and took photos of the dogs so that we would know they were okay.

There were thousands of members and many more people hoping and praying who weren't registered. It was a giant virtual waiting room where people could share their thoughts and reminisce while waiting for news.

BK: Lil, ever since the day you were born you have been a fighter! There hasnt been an obstacle in your life that you havent been able to overcome, I know for a FACT that you can and will overcome this. Thousands of people are with you, holding your hand and awaiting your recovery. I love you Lil and am constantly sending you all my love and support. ♥

December 1, 2009 at 5:10pm ·

It was also a forum for people to share their own sufferings. Some of what they shared was heart-wrenching, but it reminded us that we weren't alone.

PNF: To the Chason family:...I lost my husband on 11-15-09 ... after a 35 day stay due to H1N1...My prayers and thoughts go out to you and your family during this time...keep the faith...

December 8, 2009 at 9:55pm

It was strange that her illness was becoming such a public event. People following her story but who didn't know her, attracted by the suspense of finding out if she would get better. People cheering her on and hoping she would win, like a sporting event. But to us, it was our whole world hanging in the balance.

In the very worst case, it attracted some weird people. We received one message from an evangelical in Alabama who said, "Don't pull the plug" and that he was coming to sing by her bedside. He even called the NSICU and spoke to Cate, who said she had never talked to someone who felt so creepy. We removed his post from the site and told the security people at the hospital about it. After that, the guards were much more vigilant about checking security badges at the front desk of the hospital at night.

We let ourselves be guided by trying to think about what Lil would want us to do. We kept posting because we figured that she would be happy to know that so many people were interested in her and following her progress. We could show it to her when she was better so she could see how much she meant to people.

The hardest part for me was writing updates about her condition. There were so many ups and downs that it was tough to know when to write. I didn't even try to let people know all the details. It was too difficult. So I tried to wait until she was stable before I wrote anything.

When we didn't post for a while, the anxiety became obvious:

> CF: Can't stop thinking about Lil and the family. would love to get an update if anyone has recent info!
>
> December 1, 2009 at 6:00pm •

> LP: I did go over today and they had left the hospital for a while, so I took my little package over to the RM house. I wish I had some news, but I don't..Praying so hard!
>
> December 1, 2009 at 6:12pm •

> NHS: Thanks. we'll just wait and see what a posting brings this evening. Thank heavens for RM house. Great to hear from those of you on the ground. Sending lots of care and support to you from Rhode Island.
>
> December 1, 2009 at 6:35pm •

And later that evening:

> LP: I cannot go to sleep without knowing how Lillian is doing..Prayers continue.
>
> December 1, 2009 at 9:28pm

Anytime I mentioned even the smallest step forward, there was a flood of comments about how she was starting to get better. Even though her tidal volumes hadn't grown and the X-rays didn't show any improvement. We knew she still had a long way to go. But the people on Facebook couldn't appreciate that.

Monday 11/30 – Monday night will be one week that you have been on ECMO. They keep sending samples off to the lab to look for infection. So far, nothing has come back positive, so they are still unsure of the source of your sickness. They call what you have ARDS (adult respiratory distress syndrome). It's really a catchall phrase, since it describes the phenomenon of lungs that are stiffened by secretions and fluid buildup, but it doesn't identify the source of the inflammation. It could be H1N1, or other viruses, or probably a host of other things that I haven't heard mentioned. They are testing you for everything, so we now know that you DON'T have many things such as Lupus or many bacterial infections.

I looked up ARDS on Wikipedia. It showed an X-ray of a lung with ARDS and it looked much better than what yours look like. So now I realize the extreme severity of what you have.

The key now is patience and waiting; they are trying everything that they think will help but don't want to do too much and work against your body's own healing mechanisms.

Based on what he had been reading, Dr. Charles decided to do a few more things. He started giving Lil large doses of steroids, which have the effect of suppressing the immune response and thus help to turn off the inflammation. He had the nurses turn her over onto her stomach (called "proning") on Monday evening to give her lungs a chance to drain. This was a major production since there were so many tubes going into her body and it took a whole team of nurses to do it. She was left on her stomach all night and they flipped her back on Tuesday morning. Perhaps some slight improvement occurred, but it didn't last.

He also had them begin giving her bovine surfactant to coat the inside of the lungs and make them more slippery. It's the same treatment that they give to premature newborns whose lungs aren't able to function on their own yet. Dr. Charles mentioned that it was very expensive stuff and I asked if he had encountered any resistance to using it.

"No," he laughed. "This is just a drop in the bucket compared to everything else."

She received the first dose of surfactant on Monday morning, after they performed another bronchoscopy. We were allowed to watch, and were amazed to see how good her lungs looked. Pink and healthy, no mucous or redness as I would have expected in such a sick person.

But Dr. Charles wasn't surprised. The inflammation was occurring at the very smallest level where it couldn't be seen. He suctioned out some secretions and they looked pretty clear (and luckily didn't show a lot of blood).

Although Dr. Charles had a lot of other duties, he stopped by Lil's room often during the day. She was his only patient on ECMO and clearly his priority. Lil was only the 16th ECMO patient who had been admitted to the UNC program, which was new and understaffed, so there weren't really any other doctors to help him.

At our first meeting, he told us he would be completely in charge of Lil's care. If we had any questions, we should ask him directly and he gave us his personal cell phone number. He had smiled, then, and said we would get to know each other very well.

He'd often stand at the foot of her bed, looking at her, his arms cradled around the clipboard he always carried. I tried not to bother him with too many questions, but he never seemed to mind.

We may have been able to talk to him more easily than some families because we understood the issues pretty well from the medical/scientific point of view. But he was never arrogant or unwilling to explain why he did things or what he was thinking. It is especially rare to find this combination of skills in a surgeon: being able to make difficult decisions, understand all the medicine and still talk to patients and their families.

He was very fit and stylish. We told him we would get him on the cover of GQ when Lil got better. There was always a smile on his face and he talked easily with the nurses and technicians. It was clear that they respected and admired him by the way they talked about him when he wasn't there.

Not the type of person to give up easily, he told us multiple times that he was totally committed to Lil's getting better. But he was also honest when things were difficult, like when they found the blood in her breathing tube.

We learned a lot about his background over the course of many afternoons. He was born in Nigeria where his father had also been a doctor. His father started out as a pediatrician but then opened a hospital in the capitol, Lagos, which the family still owned and ran. The most profitable part had turned out to be the morgue that they added to it. His mother, who still lived in Nigeria, kept asking him when he was going to come home to run it. His brother had taken charge, instead, and his sister was now a pediatrician in the UK.

After opening the hospital, his father became head of the health services in Africa for the Guinness brewing company. (He said their slogan was unbeatable: "Guinness is good for you.") It was easier for Guinness to open up their own health facilities than to try to use the local health care.

Because of this, he and the other siblings went to private school in Ireland for their education. Most of the other students were the children of British families who had come to work in Ireland and it had been a pretty big cultural shock for him and his family. But one classmate's father had spent time in Nigeria in the merchant marine and they adopted him unofficially into the family. He spent all his vacations with them and still visited regularly.

After high school, he went back to Nigeria to get his medical training, then followed it up with a surgical residency in the UK and another in Los Angeles. His original plans were to become a colorectal surgeon and live a comfortable American life. He already had a job lined up at a private suburban hospital after he finished a fellowship at the University of Michigan. But during the fellowship, he learned ECMO and fell in love with the challenge of this kind of medicine, on the cutting edge between survival and death.

His wife, Celeste, grew up in NJ but is also from Nigeria originally. One of his relatives set them up at a party in the UK. She was still getting used to being in the south, a big shock after living in LA. They had a son and a daughter, both in elementary school.

Dr. Charles' attitude was always about moving forward. I had never seen this kind of leadership before and it clearly inspired all those who worked for him to be better, to try to live up to his standards. Each time he came to the ICU, he would be talking about the next move he would make and how it would improve things. I never heard him make excuses or second guess his decisions or apologize for not knowing something. Failure or incompetence was just not part of his character. He had dedicated himself to knowing all he needed to in order to do the job in front of him. He wanted to be the one responsible for making the decisions, the one with the ball.

I often thought of how much he and Lil would like each other.

Chapter 13

As a rule, my attitude towards hospitals is to stay out of them. In most of my experience, things got better by themselves if you left them alone.

Cate's history was very different. She had numerous broken bones and trips to the emergency room when she was young, often from falling off her horse. In her teens, she developed severe allergies and would have died of anaphylaxis if she hadn't been in the emergency room. This was a major reason for her becoming an acupuncturist, because it was the only thing that helped.

So I had only a few other experiences with being in a hospital, except for the girls' births.

Cate became pregnant with Lillian in the summer of 1990. Aside from some morning sickness, she otherwise felt okay. We even took a trip to Colorado, where we camped and visited some natural hot springs.

In October, Cate started to feel bad, with severe diarrhea. We took her to the hospital and they were able to diagnose it as giardia, a parasitic disease. But because of her pregnancy, we found ourselves in a horrible limbo. Her ob-gyn didn't want to be responsible for treating the giardia, and her regular doctor didn't want to treat her because he didn't want to hurt the baby.

Things changed when she found a new ob-gyn who had just arrived in town. He had previously been a veterinarian in the small town of Ruidoso before going back to medical school and relocating to Albuquerque. His background with treating animals pleased Cate immensely. Because he was new in town, he had plenty of time and he wasn't afraid to take her case.

He had her admitted to the hospital. They put her in the maternity ward, but in an isolated room away from all the others. Although it was part of the hospital, the staff wasn't comfortable with treating someone who was so sick. Although they gave her IV fluids, she still became severely dehydrated, losing 11 pounds, when she should have been gaining weight. It was painful for her to see the new mothers walking around with their babies while she felt so fearful about the safety of her unborn baby.

Nobody could tell us whether the medicine that they used to treat giardia was safe for pregnant women, but he gave it to her anyway. Cate responded well to the treatment yet still ended up staying in the hospital for 10 days. After she was released, she needed even more time to recover. Eventually, she regained her strength and the baby appeared to be unharmed.

Cate went into labor early on a Saturday evening. Her mother, Tootsie, had already come so she could be there to watch Hannah while we were at the hospital. The hospital told us we didn't need to rush, so we didn't get there until around midnight.

Cate's friend, Dorothy, came with us to the hospital to help with the birth. Walking was more comfortable for Cate than sitting, so the three of us ambled up and down the hallways all night. Her arms were wrapped tightly around Dorothy and me on each side of her as she shuffled along.

We kept the same arrangement when it came time for her to push, each of us by her side under her arms as she sat upright in the bed. Every time she had a contraction, she would squeeze so that Dorothy's and my head came together. Nearly touching noses, we would look into each other's eyes as we waited for the contraction to subside, mouthing words of encouragement.

Lillian was born at 6:05 a.m. on the 3rd of March. They didn't give her to Cate after she was born, however, as there had been some merconium staining and the nurses needed to clear out Lillian's airways. Then they took her straight to a respirator in the neonatal ICU.

"Go with her!" Cate shouted at me as they took her away.

Lillian was in the NICU for several hours before the nurses finally brought her to Cate. I stayed until things looked stable, then I went home to see Hannah and Tootsie. I brought them back to the hospital the next afternoon so that Hannah could meet her sister. She insisted on holding her and singing to her, while we hovered nearby to make sure she didn't drop her.

The following morning, I was doing errands to get the house ready—buying balloons, getting milk, etc. before going to pick up Cate. When I got back home, I found that Tootsie had been trying desperately to reach me (this was in the time before cell phones).

Cate was distraught when I called, as Lillian had suddenly gone limp while Cate was nursing her. She had run to the nurses' desk with Lil in her arms and fortunately, the pediatrician had been there. They immediately took Lillian to the NICU and put her in an incubator. She recovered her normal color after a little while with no drastic interventions.

I drove to the hospital immediately, knowing they wouldn't be coming home that day. When I got there, Lil was sleeping in Cate's arms. She seemed fine, giving no indication as to what had gone wrong. But we wanted to find out what had happened, and the reason, before we took her home.

The doctor set up several meetings with specialists to figure it out. One used a Doppler ultrasound machine that could visualize the blood flow in her heart. This was a new technique that could detect if there was a hole in the wall of her heart. In the past, they would have had to do open-heart surgery to find out, so this was a huge improvement. The technician ran the sensor over her tiny chest and we could see her beating heart on the monitor. The colors in the blood indicated the direction of the flow and there were no abnormalities.

The next day, we met with a genetic specialist. He did a bunch of simple tests like dropping Lil a small distance and catching her to observe her response and holding up her arms and watching as they fell. These seemed silly, but the doctor said they would indicate a large number of possible genetic syndromes.

We were relieved that her responses to all the tests were normal, but it didn't explain why she had lost consciousness.

The pediatrician said she couldn't explain it, but she had seen it maybe one other time. It was like the child was halfway between born and unborn, like she was trying to decide which world to be in. In her mind, it wasn't worth doing more intrusive tests if Lil didn't show any more symptoms. We should just take her home.

So we did. Cate trusted the doctor's intuition and decided not to worry. She was certain that Lillian had made up her mind to stay.

We were amazed by her calm disposition. She seldom cried or fussed. It was very different from our experience with Hannah who had been a challenge. Cate said that Lil was like an old soul. At one point, we thought maybe there was something wrong with her because she was so sweet and good.

Shortly after we returned home, I had a profound dream. I was holding Lillian when a crowd of people slowly gathered around me. They told me they had perished in the Holocaust and had never been able to have children. I said I had just had a baby and that they could love her. As I turned Lillian towards them, they surged forward wanting to take her from me. At that point, I woke up, but the cold fear of a nightmare lingered.

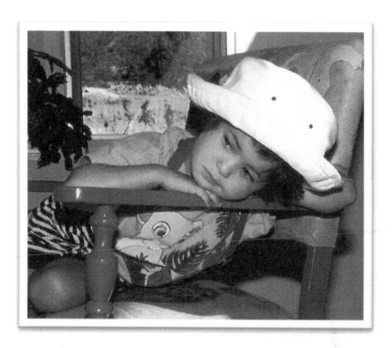

Lillian at the age of 4

Chapter 14

Tuesday, 12/1 -- I woke up about 5 a.m. and called the ICU to see how the night had gone. The nurse said you were about the same. I got to the hospital around 8:30 a.m. (after the shift change was finished). They had turned you onto your stomach again for the night and were turning you back when I arrived in the morning. So now you're on your back again as I sit here writing by your bedside.

They did another bronchoscopy in the morning and it looked about the same. They were supposed to give you more surfactant but no one could find it. The pharmacist said it may have gotten thrown out accidentally after the previous dose. They didn't have enough to give you another dose, so I was afraid they might have to put it off while they ordered some more. Since time was so important, I hated the thought of having to wait, especially if it was helping your lungs at all. The pharmacist went over to pediatrics and was able to find enough to give you another dose. It was in small packages meant for little premature babies, so they had to open a lot of them to get enough for you.

The basic plan for the rest of the day was to be patient and wait.

Cate and I had taken up very different routines. She liked to get up early and be in the hospital in the predawn hours. With only the overnight nurse and ECMO technician there, she liked the quiet time to feel close to Lil. After being in the room for a while, she would often go to the chapel to meditate, and then to the lobby to sit in the big chairs there and write in her journal. She also started writing poems that she posted on the website to share with everyone who was following Lil's progress.

I often woke up around 4 a.m. as Cate dressed. I would call the ICU to get a progress report, then fall back to sleep until about 6.

Cate took the car, so Hannah and I would wait for the first shuttle over to the hospital, which didn't come until 8:30. There was a computer at the Ronald MacDonald house, so I could read my email and check the Facebook page before having some breakfast. I often saw Cate's poems before I saw Cate. On this morning, she wrote:

> You now spin and whirl in your beautiful body
> Full of needles and tubes as big as garden hoses
> That pump your blood out into clear plastic tubes for all of us
> to see.
>
> For eleven days cocktails of ammunition have flowed through
> your veins,
> Now that war is over,
> Your body a battlefield laid bare,
>
> We wait for cool spring rains to push out anything tender and
> green.
> Anything green.
> Like miracles we do not bother to see,
> Miracles that surround us even now.
>
> You are victorious in battle.
>
> Now my Dear,
> There is time to win back your precious body, your life.
>
> Now my sweetheart
> You are a dance of light music,
> toe tapping,
> soft shoeing,
> spins and whirls,
> That special dance that always ends in a dip.
>
> We all jump out of our chairs for your ovation.
> Dear Lillian.

Cate liked to go for long walks around the campus between the spans of time she spent with Lil. I preferred to stay in the room, sometimes writing in my journal or reading the newspaper. I didn't like to miss any opportunity to see Dr. Charles or the other doctors, to hear what they were thinking. Hannah split her time between us, often walking with Cate. She didn't try to do any of the schoolwork she was missing. There would be time for all of us to get caught up when Lil was out of the woods.

When I was in the room, I watched the numbers on the ventilator constantly, hoping to see the volume start to rise as Lil's lungs started to expand. It reminded me of what I told my graduate students: "Don't watch the data as it comes into your experiment, because you can't control it, and it will be whatever it will be. It isn't up to us to get the data we want, but to understand the data we get."

Now, however, I wanted desperately to be able to control the numbers. I wanted my hoping and praying to make them start to rise. I kept staring at them, looking for the first indication that they were getting better. But I knew that these data had lots of fluctuations, and there would have to be a significant change before I could believe there was any real improvement.

9:30 p.m. Wednesday, 12/2 – It's Wednesday evening. They rolled you onto your back earlier, after you had been on your stomach all day. They also gave you surfactant.

You tolerated the rollover well, but now your blood pressure is high, shooting up to 190/120 at times. It seems frighteningly high, but the nurse doesn't seem too worried. Because you are 18, she says you can handle it. They've given you a drug to lower it, but it hasn't settled you down yet. It's hard to watch while your heart races, but she says they don't want to overreact and lower your blood pressure too much.

When your blood pressure goes up, your oxygen 'sats' go down. It was around 80 before they turned you over, but now it has dropped to near 70. Your tidal volume is the same that it's been all day.

In the evening, Lillian often had periods when her heart would start racing and her blood pressure would spike to high levels. When you looked at her lying motionless, you couldn't tell anything was wrong, but the numbers on the monitor told a different story. Her heart rate shot up to more than 170 beats per minute (from the normal value of 72). I couldn't imagine what that would feel like—I don't think I have ever gotten my heartbeat to go that fast. Her blood pressure rose to 190/120, compared to a normal of 120/80. Sometimes, the top number climbed over 200. They tell you to go see your doctor if it goes over 140! It was like watching the gauges on a sports car go into the red-zone. How long could this go on before the engine exploded?

Yet the nurses seemed unperturbed. They would calmly go over to the machine and turn off the beeper that was warning them something was wrong. They put drugs into her IV line to bring her blood pressure down, but these took a while to work. As they waited for the numbers to drop, they didn't show any sign of emotion or concern. It was better not to overmedicate, they told me, or then they would have to use other drugs to bring it back up.

I wanted to scream at them: "Can't you see what distress she's in? Why don't you do something?" But I didn't want to jeopardize the good relationship we had. So I'd tactfully ask leading questions, like, "Don't you think you should give her a little more now?"

They'd nod, as if they were considering what I said, but then they'd continue the same protocol they were already following. What would it take for them to get worked up? I wondered. What if it had been someone they loved lying in that hospital bed?

I learned from them that low blood pressure was a much bigger concern. Lil was young and healthy. Her heart could handle this extra exertion. But when the blood pressure dropped, that could be the sign

of serious complications such as sepsis or infections. Then the options
for treatment were much more limited.

Chapter 15

When Lillian was six years old, we moved into a new house outside of Albuquerque. Up until then, we had lived down in the valley, by the Rio Grande River.

The new house was in the Sandia Mountains, on a steeply sloping piece of wooded land that faced away from the city. From the upstairs windows, we could see the mountains and the fertile Estancia plain beyond it, spreading east toward Moriarty. It was a beautiful site filled with pinon trees and junipers and ancient-looking cedars. Because it was the high desert, there was no ground cover and the sandy soil was easily washed away. Deep culverts all over the property showed where the water ran when the rains came.

The builder had carved a flat circle out of the hillside for the house to be built on, but hadn't put in any retaining walls. I was afraid that without them, the dirt would wash away and return to its natural slope over time. We were house-poor, so we didn't have any money to hire someone to build them, or even to buy material for building them. But every day, they were cutting new roads for more houses and there were literally tons of rock being excavated every week and left by the side of the road.

"Do you want to collect rocks with me?" I asked Lil one Saturday afternoon in the fall. It was just the two of us at home. Cate and Hannah were off doing errands.

"Yeah!" she said immediately. I would have been surprised if she had said no. Six-year-old girls are agreeable and fun and eager to do anything with their fathers.

Several weeks before, I had gone up to the head of the road crew to ask if I could take some.

"You want this rock?" he asked me with one of those looks of amusement that I was used to getting from the construction crews. I think he was surprised that I bothered asking. There wasn't anybody around on the weekends who would have stopped me. "It's okay with me. We're just going to have to haul it off."

From then on, every chance I got, I'd put our two dogs in the back of my beat-up Ford Ranger and drive along the new dirt roads to where they were digging. I would scramble over the large piles, looking for rocks that were solid, not crumbly, and not too heavy for me to lift. I'd carry these to the truck and throw them in the back until the springs sagged so much it couldn't take any more. Then I'd bring them home and dump them alongside our driveway until I could use them.

It had become a bit of an obsession and the pile was getting pretty big. Cate had even taken to calling me "Rock." But I continued to haul as much as I could, since there were a lot of steep slopes that needed holding back. It was great exercise, and it was saving us money, a combination that I found impossible to resist.

I discovered that I had a talent for building stone walls. I would stand in front of the pile for a long time, sizing up the different candidates until I found just the right one to fill in the hole in the wall that I was building. I prided myself on doing very little cutting to fit. Instead, I got to know the shapes I had as if they were jigsaw puzzle pieces, keeping them in my mind until I had just the right place to put them.

I was building the latest wall around our small piece of flat backyard. Without a retaining wall, it would fill in over time as the rains washed it away. The exposed earth was all soft dirt called caliche, the kind that mixed up into a sticky mess when it got wet. If you walked out in it after a rain, it would stick to your boots until you were walking on six-inch platforms.

It was fun to build, like a kid in a sandbox but with 50-pound stones to play with. I designed it as I went along, adding flat areas for benches to sit on that I would later cover with flagstone. In other places, I left open sections that could be filled with topsoil and used for planters. With a little organic matter and enough water, flowers grew abundantly, releasing the life that was locked in the soil by the stingy natural rainfall. The centerpiece would be an open fireplace so we could sit out under the stars in the cool evenings, savoring the smell of burning pinon wood.

I called our Australian shepherds, Louie and Gracie, and pointed toward the truck. Louie ran and jumped over the side and into the bed in one graceful bound. Gracie, the smaller one, used the bumper to climb in more gingerly. I leaned down to pick up Lil and she threw her arms around my neck so I could lift her into the cab and strap her into her booster seat. The dogs stuck their heads into the cab through the rear window, and she screamed in delight as they slobbered over us. As we started off, they pulled their heads out of the window and took their positions flanking either side of the cab, standing proudly and barking constantly to make sure that every living thing knew we were coming.

"We're going into a new area," I told her. "It's just been dug up and maybe we'll find some good ones."

Her eyes lit up with the excitement of an explorer venturing into new territory. The road was very rugged, and as we slowly climbed over the rocky surface, her head was thrown from one side to the other. There was a large trench dug in the middle for burying the sewer and water pipes, deeper than I was tall and as wide as the truck. I drove slowly along the edge of it, trying not to scrape the rocky wall on one side or go over the edge into the trench. Eventually it widened out into a flat area where I pulled the truck over and set the emergency brake.

I got out of the truck and the dogs jumped out after me. Lil wriggled out of her seat and into my arms. I lowered her to the ground and she climbed around on the large piles of rocks that surrounded us while I started to search the vicinity, looking for ones that would match with what I already had. Lots of rocks were too big for me to carry. Others were soft sandstone that wouldn't last over time. Most of the ones I chose were hard sandstone with the characteristic red color of the area. The best were limestone, dug from the hard bedrock of the mountain, but these were less common. I could imagine the curses of the road crew when they hit one of these sections, having to slowly chisel their way through it. "One man's meat … " I thought as I gratefully gathered them for my collection.

When I found a rock I liked, I would lift it carefully, making sure I could handle it without hurting myself. Having had one back operation in my 20s, I tried to keep my perspective. The rocks may have been saving us money but they weren't worth hurting myself over. I had noticed with pride, though, that the rocks I was bringing home were getting bigger since I had started collecting them.

After a while, Lil got tired of exploring and climbed back into the open cab. She stood on the middle of the bench seat with her arms spread out over the top of it, looking out at me through the windshield. When I came near the truck, I could hear her as she talked to herself, happy to be on such an adventure.

I was getting into a pleasant rhythm of searching and hauling. The dogs jumped easily up and down the steep slopes, making circles around me like the protective shepherds they were. Each trip, Lil would comment on what I brought back. She would often name them (eagle-face, lumpy, blockhead) as I walked past her and dumped them in the back with the others.

One time, when I looked back to check on her, I could tell that she was singing to herself because when she got to the end of a song, she would shake her head as she held the last note, something that she thought all the best singers did. At home, that's how we knew when to applaud.

The truck bed could only be filled half-full before the weight was too much for the springs. But it was only filled to half of that when I dumped one more stone in and started back up the hill. I was a dozen feet away when I heard a click that made me turn back to look.

The truck was rolling backwards, towards the open trench with Lil still inside the cab.

It took me a moment to realize what was happening, then I ran for the truck as it started to pick up speed.

Lil looked at me with complete serenity. If she realized that the truck was moving, it didn't seem to bother her.

I was having trouble getting over the rough ground as the truck moved away from me and we only had a short distance before the truck fell into the deep trench. I reached the open door on the rolling truck and was able to pull myself around it and throw myself in by grabbing the steering wheel. I got one foot on the brake while the other leg was still hanging from the truck and it stopped moving.

I looked at Lil with wild eyes, hyperventilating.

She looked back at me and smiled.

Resetting the brake, I stepped out of the cab to see where we were. The wheels had come to a halt only two feet from the edge of a steep drop.

I reached into the cab and took her in my arms and held her to my chest.

She accepted my hug with Buddha-like wisdom. I don't think she ever felt any fear. She knew her daddy would never let anything bad happen to her.

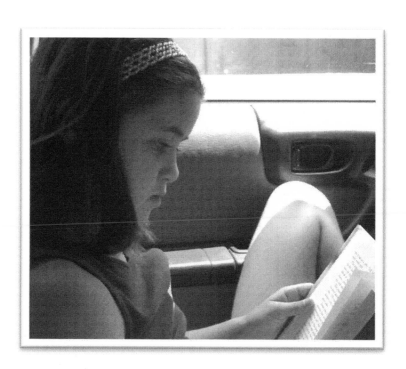

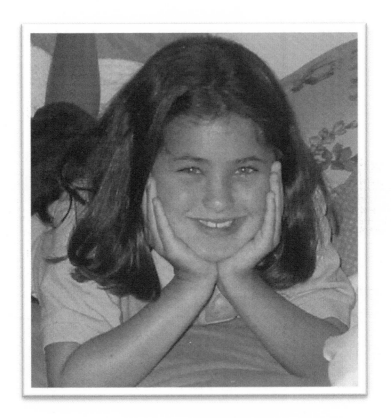

In 2001, at the age of 10

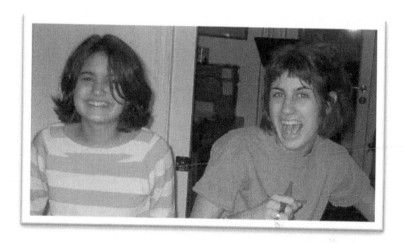

Lillian and Hannah on Hannah's 16th birthday, 2004

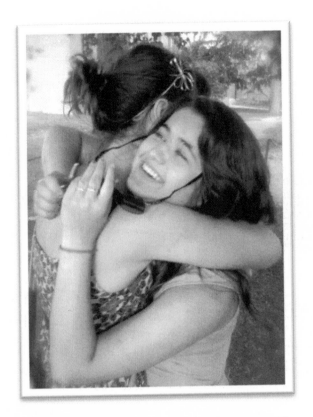

Lillian saying goodbye as Hannah starts college

Chapter 16

Thursday morning, 12/03 – It's Thursday morning and we're back in your room. Last night, you had some more extreme rises in your blood pressure. They happen pretty often—they think it may be due to lack of sedation. You are getting used to the pain-killing drugs and they also get removed by the ECMO machine. The pharmacist says you are receiving enough to stop an elephant, but still you have these periods where your heart races and the upper number on your blood pressure rises as high as 200. It takes a while to get you back down to normal each time and it is hard for us to watch because it feels like you are anxious during these periods.

When we arrive in the morning, your numbers were about what they were when we left last night—oxygen saturation around 78-80 and tidal volume around 90 mL. The tidal volume is what Dr. Charles keeps hoping will increase. It will be a sign that your lungs are becoming less stiff.

Kathy Short is going to put a humidifier back in your air line to see if it can help break up the secretions, the same way we used to turn on the hot shower and sit with you when you had the croup.

I spent a lot of time standing by Lil's bedside, holding her hand and thinking about good times we'd had together. While staring at the monitors, I'd talk to her about them, sometimes in my mind and sometimes out loud.

I am fortunate that we had spent a lot of time together. Maybe I would have been a more successful physicist if I had spent more hours at work, but after the girls were born, it just didn't seem as important. I wanted to have a closer relationship with them than I'd had with my parents, to be able to talk to them and have them be able to talk to me. They were always included in the dinner parties we liked to throw and they were comfortable talking to adults, about movies or music or whatever was going on in their lives.

We had even more time together after Hannah went to college. Without Hannah to drive Lil to school, I got to drop her off every morning on my way to work. Those short rides in the car were a great time to hear what was on her mind. Cate was working hard seeing lots of patients so that we could pay college tuition, so I also made a lot of dinners. I loved talking to Lil while she worked on her homework and I cooked dinner.

She kept getting more interesting as she got older. We'd listen to CDs she'd made from her hours on iTunes. When she had seen a movie, she always had an interesting way of describing the relationships between the characters, or the way that the story was developed that I hadn't considered. She was a great listener. I could even talk about the physics problems I was working on and she was smart enough to grasp the essential science, as well as caring enough to ask about how I felt about it.

Whenever we had to go to an eye doctor appointment, we always went to a movie afterwards. They usually dilated her eyes and it was hard for her to be in the sunlight. Sitting in a dark theater was the most comfortable thing to do, even if she couldn't really see the screen. We usually went to corny chick flicks where we could enjoy getting lost in the improbable feel-good plots, waiting for the boy and the girl to overcome some conflict or misunderstanding before the inevitable happy ending. Sitting next to her in the dark theater, hearing her laugh, seeing the big smile on her face, let us escape from any other concerns we had.

1 p.m. Thursday, 12/03 – Your blood pressure still rises, as if you are trying to wake up. You were also moving your head and it looked like you were swallowing. These are all signs to us that you want to shake this off and wake up. We talk to you and tell you that it isn't time to try breathing on your own and that you need to rest. But it doesn't help—it isn't your conscious mind that is struggling. It is something deeper.

The local TV station contacted the hospital and wants to talk to us. We told them we wouldn't talk to them now because I want to see some signs of improvement before we do. We all agree that we want them to focus on you and not on the suffering of the family.

During the afternoon, there was a period of quiet and I thought of how I used to sing to you when you were little. You were always so sweet and told me you loved it. I started singing songs I hadn't sung since you were little—Paper Moon; This Land is your Land; Good Night Irene. You lay there so quietly I could almost imagine that I was singing you to sleep again.

Lil's friends in Barrington got together one night during Thanksgiving break and made a stack of cards for her. They shipped them down in a big envelope and we read them to her. Another large stack came from a card-making event held by one of the fraternities. Prayer groups from all over North Carolina and from other states sent cards to let her know they were praying for her. We got cards from good friends and from people who had never met Lil but had heard about her from the news and the internet. Some were the parents of other freshman at UNC; they couldn't help writing because her sickness embodied the greatest nightmare that they could imagine for their own children.

Cate's favorite was from a little boy who drew a stick figure with the words, "Get up, Lillian." We pasted them up on the walls at first, but there were soon too many and we only put up selected ones.

There was a wide windowsill and Cate set up a display on it of things that people had sent. It was behind Lil's bed, so it was necessary to climb over the air hoses and the tubes carrying the blood to the ECMO machine to get to it. Cate didn't mind going back there, but I hated it when she did, thinking of how horrible it would be if one of the lines got pulled out.

The items included a beautiful forest landscape painted on glass that the sun shone through in the morning. A heart-shaped prism caught the morning light. A stuffed animal in a UNC shirt watched over everything. "Homer" was back there, too, Lil's stone fetish from New Mexico in the shape of a bear that she always carried around with her. He was in the bag of things she'd had with her when she was admitted.

People sent religious objects and we added them to the windowsill like an altar. A Hindu god in the shape of an elephant took its place beside a picture of Mona with a Bahá'í prayer. A Buddhist prayer bowl made a beautiful pure tone when struck with a wooden mallet. Ornaments from different Catholic saints were hung from a "tree" used to suspend IV lines. Prayer flags and beads were hung from the other empty hooks on it. They were accompanied by a butterfly fairy from Pat Lea. Bottles of holy water were lined up beneath it.

Even better were the packages of food, especially cookies and chocolate. Cate learned an important truth about hospital staff—the nurses were addicted to chocolate. Whenever a food package came, she would grab it (after maybe letting Hannah have a bite) and parcel it out to the different nurses stations, in the ICU and back in pediatrics where Lil had first been. She got them conditioned—whenever she walked in, they were expecting that she might have something good with her. It was never hard to get their attention if she needed something. To be less flippant about it, she was glad to share it with them. We had incredible admiration for these hard-working women and men and loved to be able to give something back to them.

There was a lot of activity on Facebook with more than 300 new posts a day offering encouragement and prayers. We could see the network spreading out as people explained how they had heard about it. Using our phones, we would step out to the corridor to read the new comments that had been posted. We heard similar things from our friends, how they couldn't stop checking the website constantly during the day to see if anything had changed and to share the warmth of all the people who cared about Lil. One friend told us he went to the Starbuck's in Barrington. Someone recognized him as a friend of ours and everyone in the shop wanted to know what he knew. We were amazed by all this interest from so many people. We said over and over how cool it would be for Lil to see this when she got better.

10 a.m. Friday, 12/4 -- We're waiting for Dr. Charles to come in and do another bronchoscopy. Yesterday you seemed very close to consciousness. Cate was here all that afternoon and visited by Leslie, Mark and Azi. They talked to you a lot and it seemed to help you remain calm. You were actually moving your eyebrows and toes and Cate felt like you were very present. Dr. Cairns (head of the burn unit) came in with Dr. Charles and he said you were clearly very special. He also said he thought you would make it, which was amazing since he is usually pretty reserved.

Overnight, your blood pressure went way down for a while. Cate called at 5 a.m. and felt like you needed someone with you so she came into the hospital. I got here at around 8:30 a.m. on the shuttle.

On Friday afternoon, we were sitting around Lil's room and getting a little punchy. It had been a long, quiet day with no new progress.

Then bizarre questions started to come up. For some reason, Cate asked Dr. Charles if he could dance.

He said he liked to salsa dance, and she told him he had to dance for us when Lil got better.

He upped the ante and said he would break dance! So we posted a photo of the ventilator's monitor screen on Facebook and told everyone that Dr. Charles would dance if the tidal volume reached 300 mL. After that, we would receive encouraging Facebook messages from everyone who was looking forward to his performance, telling her to get better so Dr. Charles could dance:

> "G'night Lil...sweet dreams and in the morning lets see those numbers where Dr. Charles needs to get out his dancin' shoes. Relax and breathe..."

December 5, 2009 at 10:51pm

> For every prayer you see here there are hundreds perhaps even thousands which are being said for you. I looked at your pictures yesterday...how beautiful you are...they are...I saw that your Dr. Charles will dance when the number hits 300....so that is what I am seeing. 300! So that he can dance, you can dance we can all dance in celebration!

December 7, 2009 at 4:22am ·

> Still praying for you Lil. Come on Dr. Charles. Get the dancing shoes ready. The whole world is waiting to see that video of you Dancing when Lil gets better. As she will.

December 7, 2009 at 5:07pm

It was like living in parallel universes. There was the reality of us being in the ICU every day, standing alongside Lil and focusing all our attention on her, hoping constantly for her condition to improve.

But there were also thousands of people monitoring her progress on the web as if it was a story unfolding. I could understand how people felt that way—the constant up's and down's, the drama.

Only for us, it was different from the script of a TV show because it was all true, and we didn't know how it would turn out.

The media had also gotten hold of the story. Lil was on the front page of the *Daily Tar Heel*, the college paper, and news spread from there. There were newspaper and television stories in Rhode Island and all over North Carolina. People would post links to the different reports on Facebook so we could watch them. Some of the media were more persistent than others, calling the ICU and pretending to be family to get information, but the hospital was helpful in dealing with them for us.

We continued our policy of not talking to them because we wanted the focus to be on Lil and not us, the anxious family. So instead, they reported on the Facebook page and all the support she was getting from friends and family. This seemed okay, because we felt that Lil would want people to know about her fight to beat this virus. But we didn't want it to turn into a circus.

Saturday, 12/05 -- Last night (Friday) you had a good night. Your 'sats' were up around 80 and your blood pressure was under better control. Cate came in around 2 a.m. to be with you. She likes being with you in the early morning when it's quiet in the hospital. By the time I came in around 9:30, your tidal volume had increased to 125 mL and we thought that things were looking up. Also, your X-ray at 10 a.m. showed some improvement—there was a lot of white, but you could see the bronchioles much clearer. But the airways still weren't extending very far into the further reaches of the lungs where they needed to be.

On the negative side, there were also lots of clots developing on the venous side of the ECMO machine. They could be seen as fibrous stripes on the inside of the tubing. The danger is that they will break off and block the oxygenator. But it is good that they now have two oxygenators on the machine so it won't be so catastrophic if one gets clogged. They could replace it without having to turn off the machine completely. The "bladder" (which is a reservoir to allow for pressure fluctuations in the circuit) also has a large clot that has been there for awhile. There aren't any clots yet on the arterial side of the machine, i.e., the side that delivers oxygenated blood back to the body. This would be serious because if they broke off, they would go into your blood system and could cause a stroke or a blockage in your lungs.

They suctioned your lungs again and got a significant amount of secretions out. But now, your volume has dropped to 115 mL and your 'sats' are below 80 again. So we aren't seeing the steady improvement that we are hoping for. We hope that you'll have a good night and show more progress.

Chapter 17

Ever since she left for college, I missed the time Lil and I used to spend together working on her schoolwork. It would often happen while I was in the kitchen preparing dinner, on the nights when Cate worked late. We have a small house and the kitchen was the only place where Lil had enough room to spread out her books in front of her. Since her eyesight had started getting worse, an assistant in the guidance office printed out her handouts and assignments in large type format so she could read them. They looked like a children's book, even though they contained college-level material, and they took up a lot of space.

Reading assignments, like literature and social studies, she could do upstairs in her room. She got special audio books for these subjects that could be read with a device designed for the visually impaired. It allowed her to speed up the playback—once she got used to it, she would listen to her reading assignments at several times the normal speed. It sounded like an info-commercial announcer on speed, but she could understand it. To keep from losing her concentration, she started knitting while she listened. I would often walk by her room and see her sitting on the bed propped up by her pillows, with her big earphones on, listening to her homework while her needles clicked away.

But this wasn't possible with math and science, where she needed to be able to see the equations and figures, so she spread out on the island in the kitchen. She sat in a stool on one side, working on her homework while I stood on the other side, chopping vegetables. She often didn't need any help and we would talk about other things, like what she was listening to on her iPod. At other times, she would ask me to explain a tough concept like angular momentum, or help with a tricky homework problem. Often I could give her some additional insight into it or add an anecdote about how that idea was important for something else, like how a rocket operated.

Lil was a quick learner and enjoyed understanding things, so it was fun to work with her. I could see that little light go off in her eyes when something that hadn't made sense suddenly did. Once you really understand something, it's like common sense; you can't imagine not knowing it or it being any other way. Lots of times there isn't a big distance between confusion and understanding, but it's impossible to get there without a little guidance.

Lil often commented on how hard it was for her friends, who didn't have someone like me to explain it to them.

"It's okay if your friends want to call me with homework problems," I told her.

"That would be pretty weird," she said as she shook her head. Her facial expression showed that she marveled at how clueless I could be.

On the other hand, when she didn't understand something, it wasn't pretty. One evening in the spring, I was at the kitchen counter cleaning up after dinner. She came down from her room and asked if I could help her with her calculus homework. It's not important what it was, but she just didn't get it (for those who care, it was about parametric equations, where the x and y variables each depend on a third independent variable). I tried explaining it to her in several different ways to help her understand. I explained how it was an important concept in physics, where the third variable could be time and the x and y could be positions in space.

I remember this taking a while to sink in when I learned it, so I wasn't surprised she was having trouble. But she was getting more and more frustrated as we talked. I made a cardinal mistake by saying, "Relax, it just isn't that hard."

"Why do you say that?" she screamed back at me. "I just don't get it."

"You're not listening to what I'm saying," I answered back, apparently too smugly.

"You always talk down to me," she said. "You act like this stuff is so easy."

"I've been doing this for a long time," I said. "It makes sense to me. But that doesn't mean I think it's easy to learn."

"Why do you always treat me like I'm so stupid?"

This caught me by surprise. First of all, it wasn't true. I thought she was an amazing student. But it hurt to know that she thought I patronized her. I wish that I had said nothing, but I couldn't stop the feeling of anger that was rising in me.

"I can't believe you said that to me," I shouted back at her. "I do not talk down to you. You're just mad because you don't understand it and you're blaming me."

She stopped and started to cry, holding her head in her two hands, staring down at the counter. "How am I going to be able to do this myself?" she said.

Now I felt stupid. It was about a lot more than a few math problems. She was scared about the future, about making her way after she lost her sight. But what could I say to her?

"You'll be fine," I said, trying to downplay it, not knowing how else to console her. "Besides, I'm going to move into the dorm room next to yours."

She continued to look down and she just shook her head.

"You can't learn anything when you're angry," I said. "Go do something else for a while."

Lil closed her books without saying anything else and went upstairs to her room.

I finished cleaning up and went to my study to answer some emails and prepare for my next lecture.

When Cate came home, I had a glass of wine with her while she had a bite to eat. Around 10, I went upstairs to go to bed, passing Lil's open door at the end of the hallway. She was at her desk working at her computer. It was a machine designed specially for her with an extra large screen and software that allowed her to magnify any text. It also had a reading feature so that the computer would speak anything she put the cursor on. She leaned forward in her chair, her face up close to the monitor so she could see what she was working on.

I went in to give her a hug and say goodnight.

She stopped what she was doing and looked up from the screen. She had gone on to other things and showed no trace of anger from our fight earlier.

"Do you want to look at your calculus anymore?"

"No, I'll do it later. I've got to finish this paper," she answered.

I was sound asleep when I felt a small hand touch me on the shoulder. "Can you help me?" she asked.

"Yeah, I guess so," I said as I woke up. I turned around and saw the clock; it was almost 2 a.m.

We went back down the stairs to the kitchen. Her books were spread out and it looked like she had been working for a while. She picked up the homework assignment and pointed to a problem.

"Can you do this one?"

I stared at the page for a few minutes to clear my mind and try to understand what it was asking. I had that strange feeling that you get when you're between asleep and awake. *I always said I could do this in my sleep*, I thought to myself.

After it made sense, I restated the problem to Lil to help her understand it.

She took in everything I said calmly, nodding her head. Then she started to write.

The kitchen was quiet, the silence only offset by the sound of the refrigerator humming and her pencil scratching over the paper. The cool night air had that special smell—clean, metallic—that it only has when you wake up really early. It reminded me of when we would leave for family vacations, getting up before dawn to get a jump on the driving. We would carry the girls to the car in their pajamas and let them sleep, then wake them for breakfast after we'd gone a few hours.

"Is this right?" she asked, showing me her work.

I looked over what she had done. "Yes," I said.

I felt like I was sharing a piece of Lil's life that I usually missed. While we were upstairs asleep she was often down here working until early in the morning. The cool air, the complete quiet—it was like being transported to another world. I used to live in this world when I was a college student, embracing the stillness of the night for doing my own work. But that was a long time ago, before children, before schedules, before needing to wake up in the morning for meetings and classes.

We went on to the other problems that she hadn't been able to do. The explanations and hints I gave her weren't much different than what I'd tried to explain earlier. It was just that now she was able to receive it. It didn't take long to finish and after about half an hour, she said she was done.

"Go to bed," I told her as she closed up her books.

The next morning, when the alarm went off, I said to Cate, "Let her sleep. I'll call the school and tell them she'll be late."

Chapter 18

Sunday, 12/06 – Cate was here in the early morning when they came in to take your X-ray. She saw that they didn't shield your ovaries when they X-rayed you and got extremely angry. She was very mad at Dr. Charles and said that she bet he wouldn't let his own children have that many X-rays without shielding. We argued, because I thought her anger was misplaced. I agreed that they should have been shielding you (it doesn't cost anything to put a lead apron over you) but I was concerned that she not make it personal with him and ruin our good relationship.

Cate was angry and had been crying for a while by the time I got to Lil's room. She was getting one or two X-rays every day and Cate didn't understand why they wouldn't put shielding over her abdomen. Didn't they care that she might have children? Did this mean they didn't think she would survive?

The nurses called Dr. Charles, and when he arrived, he went right up to her and asked what was wrong. I was always impressed with how direct he was at dealing with things—he never shied away from facing them. I think this is especially amazing in a surgeon, because they aren't renowned for talking to people.

He suggested that Cate go for a walk with him and they were gone for two hours. Later, she told me about some of the things they talked about. He'd discussed the lack of enthusiastic support for the adult ECMO program from some of the hospital doctors. There were some people, like Dr. Cairns, the head of the burn unit, who believed in him wholeheartedly. But he was still trying to prove that it was a worthwhile technique, justifying the high cost and highly trained staff. He didn't have much backup, which is why he said we could always call him directly. There weren't other doctors with his level of training in ECMO that he could trust.

Lil's case mattered a lot to him, even beyond her own health. He had asked a colleague (not at UNC) about whether he should take our case. He mentioned that the chancellor of the university knew about Lil and that I was a Brown professor and Harvard graduate. His friend had told him he wouldn't touch it with a 10-foot pole. Luckily he'd taken it anyway. But there was clearly a lot riding on this for everyone.

He also explained to Cate that he didn't have control over the radiology department. They were not part of the ECMO team and their staff didn't answer to him. But he assured her that he would talk to the director and that Lil would be shielded whenever she got X-rays in the future.

Sunday, 12/6 -- Your numbers went down over the course of the day. The 'sats' were 88 in the morning but then dropped to 70 and haven't come up all day. But you've been relatively stable the rest of the time. Your nurse has a 15-year-old daughter and she treats you like a mother would, so you are well taken care of.

Chuck Sherman arrived at the hospital around 4 p.m. He's a good friend and also a pulmonologist, so we'd been talking on the phone every day. Earlier in the week, he said he'd come down if I wanted him to.

"I can't get anything done, anyway," he said. "I spend all my time looking at her Facebook page for updates."

We walked into Lil's room and he saw the ECMO machine for the first time. He stood there a while and appraised it, like a new car buyer in the show room. Rhode Island didn't have a single ECMO machine for adults—only for pediatrics. We were fortunate that Lil got sick in North Carolina, because not many places had this capability. God bless the competition between Duke and UNC; they'll each buy anything to stay out in front of the other.

After getting some dinner, we came back to the hospital so Chuck could meet Dr. Charles. They had been talking on the phone regularly, after Chuck asked me to find out whether he would mind talking to him. Some doctors don't want others getting involved in their cases, but fortunately Dr. Charles wasn't like many doctors (especially surgeons).

Chuck deals with a lot of patients each day, juggling a busy practice with an adjunct faculty position at the medical school. Cases like Lil's were his specialty, but he was sensitive enough to not be too pushy. "I'll be a lamb," he promised. "And if I have any ideas, I'll make sure Dr. Charles thinks they're his."

They were both involved in health projects in Africa and they knew some of the same people. Chuck shared some information about potential granting agencies and I could see how appreciative Dr. Charles was. It was easy to forget that he was still a young doctor, early in his career, trying to establish a reputation for himself.

Listening to them talk, it was good to know that they were in agreement about Lil's treatment. I couldn't imagine how much harder this would be if we didn't have faith in our doctors. Every option they discussed was about risk vs. benefit. What would it help and how could it hurt? Most of the decisions had to be made with only incomplete information, so I was especially impressed at how Dr. Charles never seemed to second-guess himself. He didn't obsess over whether what he was doing was right. He made the best decision he could with the available information, and if there were complications, he dealt with them as they came up. Always moving forward. Very unlike the kind of science I do, where we analyze things to death until we fully understand them. Of course, when my students make a mistake, nobody gets hurt.

After Dr. Charles left, Chuck and I stayed in the room and talked for a while. After seeing her X-rays, he said there was no question in his mind that she needed to go on ECMO.

But why weren't her lungs opening up? She didn't seem to have symptoms of the flu anymore.

The problem, Chuck explained, was at the smallest level, in the alveoli, tiny sacks at the furthest end of the air passageways. They were filled with secretions and had to pop open to become functional.

Later, I posted on the Facebook page that her lungs needed to open like lilac blooms in the spring. When I looked back later, several people had put up pictures of lilacs opening up, exactly what I had envisioned when I wrote it. The invisible community of people following Lil's progress, eager to do anything they could to help. Beside one picture, it said:

> "Goodnight Lillian, rest well tonight and in the morning may the blooming begin. We are beside you every step..."

Chapter 19

Monday, 12/07 – You had a quiet night. By the time we left your room on Sunday, you were well sedated and our goal was to let you try to regain some ground. Overnight, your tidal volume rose to 130 mL when Cate came in to see you around 3 a.m. You had been on ECMO for 2 full weeks, so Dr. Charles asked us to all meet to discuss our options.

We got together on Monday morning at 7 a.m. in the same little conference room where, two weeks earlier, we had been asked to put Lil on ECMO. Hannah and I came in from the Ronald Macdonald House and got Cate out of the ICU, where she had been by Lil's bedside since the early hours of the morning. Chuck walked over from the Carolina Inn where he'd spent the night. Dr. Charles had also asked the head of nursing and some other members of the ECMO team to be there. He came in and got started right away.

"I wanted you all to be here together so there aren't any questions about what is going on," he said. The previous week had had no major difficulties but also no major progress. Progress meant significant increase in her tidal volume, the useable volume of the lung as it expands when you breathe in. She needed them to get less stiff, to get big enough so she could survive without ECMO. A normal, healthy person had a volume of around 500 mL. Lil's was around 100. It had to get to be at least 250 mL before she had a chance.

And then he calmly said that if Lil wasn't making progress by next Monday, we would have to stop ECMO.

This wasn't what I expected. He had never talked about stopping before. His focus was always on what to do next. I started to protest, but he continued, making it clear this wasn't something to be discussed or argued about. He was just laying out the facts. If she was making progress and wasn't there yet, he would continue to support her. But Lil couldn't be on ECMO indefinitely and if she weren't getting better by next week, the chances of improvement would be disappearing.

I looked around the room. Cate and Hannah didn't say anything. Chuck just nodded his head, the nurses and technicians nodding along with him.

I felt so alone, like I was the only one who heard him, who understood what this meant. Everyone else seemed so detached, so absorbed in their own thoughts.

"So, it's time to make some big moves," Dr. Charles said breaking into a large smile. He was warming up, now that he could talk about doing something. The ECMO machine needed to be changed out again because it was beginning to develop clots. Although Lil might be starting to heal, if they didn't replace the machine, it was likely that it would fail before she could get off of it. The new machine would be fit with dual oxygenators to keep them from cracking again. To suppress the allergic reaction that caused her to swell up so badly, they would use a new approach and prime the new machine with blood instead of saline solution. This should allow her to recover more quickly and reduce the time to accommodate to the change in machine.

He paused before he got to the next item. "I also want to insert a second canula in her leg, on the other side of her groin." The canulae were the stiff tubes that brought the blood into Lil's body. All along, the staff had been battling with the fact that they could only get a small flow out of the machine because the canulae were too small, because Lil was small. They had to use high pressures that made the oxygenators crack. A second canula would let them increase the flow and give them better ability to control the blood oxygenation.

The risk of putting it in was just like when they first put her on the machine. They would have to blindly snake the tubing up through her groin toward the heart, without being able to see where it was actually going. If it caused bleeding internally, they wouldn't be able to stop it because of all the blood thinning heparin that she was getting. If this happened, she would die. On the plus side, he said, Lillian is a healthy 18- year-old girl with nice, smooth veins that have a lot of resiliency. As always, it was a balance of risk and benefit.

What could we say? It was one more hurdle we would have to leap over. We had to put our faith in Dr. Charles. There was no other way to go. And he showed no lack of certainty that this was the right thing to do.

He wanted to get started right away. The ECMO machine kept her from being moved, so they would do the procedure right there in Lil's room. Since he could do it himself, he didn't have to wait for others to schedule it. He smiled as he left the conference room to get suited up. These challenges were exciting to him.

After he left, we each took up our own rituals for waiting. Cate couldn't bear to stand around and grabbed Hannah to go for a walk. She said to call her if anything happened. On the other hand, I wanted to stay as close as possible. Chuck said he would wait with me. "Hey man, I'm your Sherpa," he said.

We weren't allowed in the ICU while they operated, so we stood in the corridor, leaning against the concrete block wall that faced the ICU door.

I stared at the door, focusing all my thoughts on Lil. "C'mon, kid. You can do this." Rooting for her, hoping for her, begging her to get better. It was a familiar mental litany that had developed over the last two weeks, but now it was even more focused and intense.

The wooden door was locked and solid, with no window. Doctors and staff could swipe their cards to get in, but visitors had to wait to be buzzed in by the receptionist. It opened and closed automatically, with leisurely speed, unhurried and not to be rushed.

Every time someone came in or out, I craned my head around them to look into the ICU. Lil's room was at the end of the straight corridor, past the receptionist's desk, surrounded by closed curtains. The tops of the heads of the surgical team were barely visible above the fabric. I could recognize Dr. Charles by the navy blue bandanna he wore over his hair as he operated. University of Michigan colors, I thought, from where he trained.

The first thing they would do was change over from the old machine to the new one. Cate and Hannah came back while they were still working and lined up along the wall next to Chuck and me. Hannah slumped to the floor and sat looking at her knees. Cate and Chuck talked about things back in Rhode Island.

Each time the door started to open, I jumped into the middle of the hallway to get a brief glimpse into the room. The people going in and out were wrapped up in their own thoughts, oblivious of me standing on my tiptoes, staring past them.

After about an hour, a nurse came out and told us that the first stage, changing the machine, had gone okay. We were allowed in to see her briefly while they gave her body time to adjust to the new machine. The nurses cleaned up from the operation while we stood around Lil in her bed. Everything seemed as it had before, Lil resting quietly while the pumps on the machine quietly turned. Then they asked us to leave so they could put in the new canula.

We resumed our positions on the wall outside the ICU. I didn't want to talk to anyone, just keep my attention focused on the door and the brief glimpses I could get inside. It was as if, if I didn't pay enough attention, something bad would happen.

After a short time, the same nurse came out to tell us that the new canula had gone in with no complications. Relief flooded over me. I had always felt scared about this procedure, ever since Dr. Charles had first told us how difficult it was to put someone on to ECMO.

The nurse said that she would come back again after they had turned on the blood flow to the machine. She disappeared back into the ICU.

Every time the door opened, I would get another glimpse. It was calm around Lil's bedside, as far as I could see, but it all seemed to be taking a long time. Then I saw a head standing taller than all the others, leaning over her bed and bobbing up and down rapidly.

A young nurse walked through the door and Cate grabbed her and asked her what was happening.

She was clearly uncomfortable. "I don't know," she stammered. "I'm not working on her. I can't tell you."

Then she wheeled around and went right back into the ICU. After a moment, she came back and told us that we should go to the conference room and wait for Dr. Charles to come talk to us.

No one moved. There was no way we were going to leave the spot where we were standing.

Dr. Charles finally came out. Lil's heart had stopped when they'd started the blood flowing into the new canula. They had been doing CPR on her for approximately 20 minutes and her heart wouldn't resume its normal rhythm. "I don't think she is going to make it," he told us, and said we could come in to say goodbye.

Without a word, Cate walked past him and marched into the ICU with the rest of us following.

A half-dozen nurses and doctors surrounded her bed. The scene seemed weirdly familiar, like one from a hundred hospital TV shows. One doctor held the electrical paddles to her chest to restart her heart, and her body jumped when they pulsed it.

But the line on the monitor wouldn't come back.

Cate, Hannah and I went straight up to Lil, pushing the others out of the way.

I grabbed Lil's left hand and started talking to her, telling her that she didn't have to go, that she could come back to us.

Cate took her left foot in her hands and started pressing acupuncture resuscitation points while she called out to her.

Hannah held her other foot and begged her to hold on.

Dr. Charles went over to the nurse who was still doing CPR and told her quietly that it was okay to stop.

He turned to Cate, telling her that she needed to let go. He asked the nurses how long it had been. Lil's heart had stopped around 11:40, and it was now a few minutes after noon.

He was about to call the time of death, but Cate had a look of determination on her face that I hadn't seen since she was in labor with the girls. She looked him in the eye and said, "Not yet. She has a pulse."

The nurse standing by Lil's left shoulder agreed.

Dr. Charles reached over and felt Lil's neck. He shook his head and said it wasn't.

Then a young doctor who was staring at the monitor said he saw a heartbeat.

A nurse said dismissively that there wasn't a pulse, but the doctor stuck to his guns. "Give me a Doppler unit," he said.

There wasn't a sound around Lil's bed as he squeezed gel on her wrist and placed the probe on it. He moved it around, searching for her artery, any sign of a pulse.

Gradually, a faint whooshing sound started to come from the machine. An unreal sound. Very soft. The same sound as on the ultrasound machine in the ob-gyn's office when we heard Lil's heartbeat for the first time.

Cate kept looking at Lillian's face and said, "Don't take it off."

Nobody moved from the bedside, not the nurses, the doctors, or us. We all stared at Lil, wordlessly willing her heart to continue.

Slowly, with each beat, it got stronger.

Dr. Charles didn't say anything but just shook his head in wonder. Even though Chuck is a doctor, he said he had never seen anything like it. Eventually a normal rhythm returned.

None of us wanted to leave. We kept repeating the events to each other to convince ourselves it had actually happened. Dr. Charles had been ready to give up, but Cate, Hannah and I, we all knew. We had each felt it as we stood next to her, with our hands on her. She didn't want to go.

. . . . .

Monday afternoon -- The problem now is that they put a lot of pressure on you when doing the CPR and there is bleeding in your lungs. The breathing tube is filled with frothy red fluid. When they suction you, they get even more bright red liquid. I realize that this is what Dr. Charles was worried about when they called us to come to the hospital in the middle of the night that first week you were on ECMO.

There was no time for the team to rejoice in the miracle we had just been a part of. Dr. Charles started giving instructions to deal with the bleeding. He let us stay by Lil's bedside, even though crucial decisions needed to be made quickly.

They immediately backed down on the heparin to allow her blood to clot. Another drug was started to help with clotting. It was more important to stop the bleeding than to worry about clots building up in the machine. The pressure was increased in the ventilator to act like applying pressure to a wound. Still, there was a lot of blood when they suctioned her lungs again.

He didn't sugar coat what else they needed to do. They had to know if Lil's brain had been damaged while her heart was stopped, so he ordered them to turn off her sedation. "We might expect her to blink by around midnight," he told us, by which point the drugs would have worn off.

After all this trauma, the numbers on the monitors looked bad. Her sats had dropped down into the 40s from a high of 79 in the morning, before the operation. The results of another chest X-ray came back and showed a dark region in her lungs. In general, dark was good: the fluid-filled lungs showed up as white and opaque on the X-rays. As they cleared up, they would appear darker.

At first, Dr. Charles was very excited, until he realized that it was not clearing of the lungs, but a pneumothorax (air in the space around the lungs). Chuck, more familiar with seeing these kinds of lung problems, had already recognized it.

Dr. Charles ordered the equipment so that he could put in a chest tube to drain the air out of it as well as let out additional liquid. Chuck told me how great it was that Dr. Charles is a surgeon because he could do procedures like this himself instead of having to schedule somebody else to do it. For a trauma surgeon, putting in a chest tube is not a big deal.

Dr. Charles said he had to leave for a while to attend to other business. It was hard to remember, sometimes, that Lil wasn't his only patient. Then he would be back to put in the chest tube.

I was standing alone by Lil's bed when she started to move around. It was around 3 p.m., much sooner than we'd expected.

More than simply blink, she was trying to breathe, heaving her shoulders upwards. Then she started to kick her legs.

The nurses had to scramble to get her sedation adjusted again, but it was clear that she wasn't giving up.

We waited outside the ICU door again while Dr. Charles put in the chest tube. This time everything went smoothly and he came out to tell us. They had taken off a lot of liquid and now the lungs had room to expand again. Her sats were back up in the low 80s and Dr. Charles was happy as he said goodbye to us for the day.

Cate went back to our room to go to sleep so she could get up early and sit with Lil before dawn, when no one else was around. Hannah, who looked pretty drained, went with her.

I didn't want to leave yet, so Chuck stayed with me. He was going back to Rhode Island the next day. I stood by Lil's side, not letting go of her hand.

"You know," he said, "her sats are stable. They got her on a new machine. If you forget what happened this morning, it's actually been a pretty good day."

I smiled and just shook my head. What else was there to say?

There was no way to explain what had happened to those who hadn't been there, but I knew people wanted to know how she was doing. So when I got back to the Ronald Macdonald house, I went to post a brief update on Facebook.

I saw that Cate had posted a poem early that morning:

"Today is that day
(I humbly ask)
To Will that moment --
That spark
That intention
That cataclysmic turning
That turning of the tide
To make that decision
To be blessed

To be honored.....
As I write these words a man walks by,
Phone to his ear
And says,
"Good morning.
She has dilated 8 centimeters.
3 centimeters in the last hour!!".......

He walks rapidly,
I am no longer privy to the rest of his conversation.
It is obvious that there is new life entering this world
Now,
In this hospital.
Before this day is over
He will be a father.

18 years ago Lillian was pushed into this world.
As her mother, I pray that
Now
She find her birth again.

Listen to me.
Dilate.
Transition through that canal.

No suffering (you have had enough)

Make your birthday today.
Just remember how.
You already know your name.

The image of the pregnant woman was haunting. Cate had written it in the morning, while she was waiting with Lil, before we had even met with Dr. Charles. She couldn't know how prophetic it would be.

Chapter 20

For the first few weeks after high school ended, college was a taboo subject. The semester had been hard and Lil was worn out. Reading was getting more difficult and she was always tired from staying up late. I tried to tell her that she didn't have to work so hard now that she was already accepted to college.

"Yeah, right," she answered, not believing me. It was just too big a change in my attitude—I'd always expected her to work her hardest. In addition, she wanted to finish what she had started. She had signed up for two advanced-placement classes that continued even after some of her friends' workload had started to wane. But she refused to slow down. It infuriated her that some people thought she wasn't smart because she had a disability.

For the AP tests, she was given a large-print version of the exam and allowed time and a half because of her trouble reading the questions. After she was done with the physics test, she called me to pick her up. It was early evening—seven hours after she had started. I drove to the high school and waited in the parking area in front of the building for her to come out. As I sat in the car, buses arrived bringing the lacrosse team back from a game. The excited students leaped out of the bus, laughing and shouting to each other as they looked for their parent's cars.

Lil stepped out of the front door of the school and scanned the parking lot, searching for me. I got out of the car and waved so that she could see me, and she acknowledged me with a perfunctory nod. Her slumped shoulders showed me how exhausted she must feel.

As she trudged slowly towards the car, a mother of one of her friends intercepted her. Lil had trouble recognizing people because she couldn't make out their faces. It was one of her greatest frustrations.

But this woman knew her well and got up close. She leaned in to ask Lil how she was, not aware she was coming out of the same exam that her son had finished hours ago. They were too far away for me to hear them, but Lil's gestures told the story. I saw her throw up her hands, then she started laughing and then she began to cry.

The woman gave her an understanding smile, but I don't think she really understood how Lil was feeling.

We both got into the car and Lil just sat there shaking her head. "She must think I'm a complete nut job," she said as she sank into her seat.

"You okay?" I asked.

"Please," she said, "just take me home."

So when graduation came and school was over, Lil made it clear that she didn't want to hear about getting ready for college or anything else that smacked of education. Two Sundays after school ended, we all went over to the home of our friends Annie and Barry for brunch. Over eggs and bagels, the table littered with newspapers, we caught up on each others' lives. The talk turned to Lil, about what she wanted to do, what classes she would take, how she was going to pick her roommate.

After a few minutes, Lil exploded. "I don't even want to go to college!" she screamed and ran into the TV room, slamming the door.

"What's the matter?" Annie asked.

"Oh, she's just scared and tired," Cate tried to explain.

Through the door came Lil's voice: "Do you think I can't hear you?"

After a while, Lil allowed Annie to enter the room and talk to her, but she wouldn't share her feelings with Cate or me.

We told her she didn't need to worry about getting a job, that she could do what she wanted for her last summer at home (not adding the "you deserve it" that we were feeling).

She signed up for back-to-back morning sessions of rowing at the Narragansett Boat Club. She'd fallen in love with the sport after she had to give up softball. It was enough of a passion to make her want to get up at 7 a.m., even in the summer. In the afternoons, she came home and napped, or played with iTunes or watched her favorite TV shows on the computer.

In the evenings, she saw Matt. He would come over after he finished working at Staples. Sometimes they went out with friends, or to dinner at Bebop Burrito, but a lot of times they would just hang out at our house, never seeming to tire of each other's company.

When I came home late, the first thing I usually saw was the back of the large two-person armchair moved right up next to the TV with their heads barely visible above the top of the cushions. A big Red Sox fan, Matt often had the game on. When I asked Lil if she could see the ball, she said, "No, but Matt's using his announcer voice and telling me what happens."

On top of her daily routine, she went to the beach and a weekend at Martha's Vineyard with friends, attended the Newport Folk Festival, and spent a week at a lake in the Berkshires. Sometimes I would pick her up after rowing and we'd go to a movie to escape the sun. It was a great summer.

On the college front, she received a thick packet from UNC that she gave to me and asked me to read.

"Honey, you're the one who's going to college, not me," I said.

"Just read it and tell me what to do," she pleaded.

I looked at the many forms in small type and decided not to make an issue of it. It said that every student had to go to freshman orientation. She didn't want to make a trip down there in the summer, but as an out-of-state student, she could put it off until the week before classes started. There was also an online booklet containing course information and the Byzantine distribution requirements. It was formatted like a legal contract and difficult to read, even for me. I expanded it and printed it out for her but she never wanted to look at it, even though I asked her many times.

There was also an explanation of an unusual system they had for picking your roommate. A website allowed students to contact each other, like internet dating. This got Lil interested and she spent a lot of time online talking to potential roommates. She wouldn't talk to me about how it was going, but I overheard her talking to Cate a little about different girls who seemed interesting.

"How do I know if they're serious? I don't want to seem too eager."

In the end, the girl she was most interested in stopped writing after she told her about her visual impairment. If Lil was disappointed, she didn't let on. She said most of the students didn't end up finding a match and it was okay if they just assigned her someone.

Two nights before Lil was supposed to leave, some friends took us out for dinner, along with Matt. At the end of the meal, Lil said she had something to ask us.

"Would it be okay if Matt came over tomorrow night and stayed up to pack with me?"

Throughout high school, Lil had had a midnight curfew and so had Matt. Since she was about to be living on her own, Lil explained, couldn't we change the rules just for this one night?

Sometimes time just comes to a complete stop. I can still see that sweet, young girl leaning over her cake, her face framed by her long, brown hair, making her well- thought-out case while her boyfriend looked on, hopefully. They had clearly talked over how she was going to present this. And she was right—she would be living on her own soon.

But she had no idea how it felt to so suddenly be forced to face it, like driving over the edge of a canyon and realizing there's no turning back.

Time started again when, as usual, Cate made up her mind quickly and told her, "Sure."

Then Lil launched the second part of her plan. She wasn't surprised when we said yes, but she knew that Matt's mother would be a tougher sell.

"Could you tell her it's okay with you?" she asked.

I took a napkin and wrote on it with my red marking pen, then handed it to Lil. She read it aloud: "We give up."

"This should work," she said, smiling.

It did. The next evening, Matt came over to spend the night and help her finish her packing. Before starting, they went out with their friends. Lil was the first one of the group to leave for school so this was the first farewell. They came back after Cate and I had already gone to bed. From upstairs, we could hear the familiar sounds of her friends talking and laughing, knowing we wouldn't hear them again for a while. We could feel the emotions in their voices even if we couldn't hear the words.

I woke up at my usual 6:30 and walked downstairs to let the dogs out into the yard. Lil and Matt were sitting up on the couch in the living room, sound asleep. Their eyes were closed, but he had his arm around her and her head rested on his shoulder.

When Cate came down, we tiptoed around and let them continue to sleep while we took the dogs to the park for a walk, our typical Sunday routine. When we got home, they were awake, and so was Hannah, who was home briefly before leaving to spend her junior year in Montana. Cate made them all French toast, Lil's favorite, and then Hannah helped me finish packing the car.

Lil was in tears when we told her it was time to leave. She and Matt stood by the front door and held each other for a long time until we gently told her we had to go. She climbed into the back seat of the car, arranging the various loose bags and clothes around her to make room for herself. She looked out the window at Matt; the pain on his face was unbearable to watch. Tears rolled down his cheeks as he ran alongside the car while we slowly drove away.

Driving down I-95, we took the same route that we followed on all our summer trips to the beach in North Carolina. Those times had been filled with the excitement of starting our vacation, what Lil always referred to as the best week of the year. We would rent a van and the girls would each have their own seat to spread out in, creating their own universe. Lil would take the furthest back row and surround herself with pillows and towels, building a nest from which she could watch the road unfold. The things she would occupy herself with changed over the years. Dolls turned into Game Boys, then Walkman's and iPods, but she was always content.

This time, curled up in the back seat of our small car, headphones in her ears, she kept her eyes downcast, crying.

When we got near to the border with Connecticut, Lillian suddenly cried, "Daddy, take me home. I don't want to go." Her voice sounded like a little girl, a voice I hadn't heard for years.

"I know, Sweetie," I said. "I know."

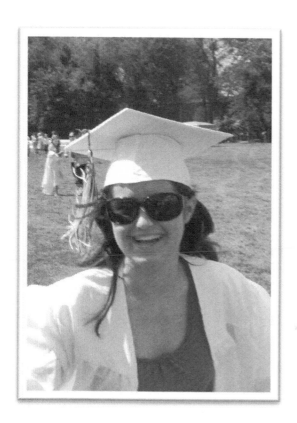

High School Graduation

Chapter 21

Around 8 p.m., we stopped driving for the night in Delaware. We went into a nearby restaurant for dinner, but Lil asked to be excused after only a few minutes. Cate and I finished eating but we weren't able to enjoy the food. When we went back to the car, Lil was in the back seat, staring at her phone, texting her friends, still with tears in her eyes. Neither of us tried to talk her out of how bad she was feeling or tell her it would all be okay. Leaving home was probably the hardest thing she'd ever done.

We arrived at Cate's cousin Melinda's house the next night, a big old farmhouse in the country outside of Chapel Hill. With two big, old dogs and chickens roosting in the trees, it reminded me of the house in Albuquerque where we'd lived when Lil was born. Having friends and family in the area was one of the things that made it possible to imagine Lil being so far away from us.

Melinda, also a UNC alum, had always looked up to her older-cousin Cate, and I think she was happy to be in a similar position for Lil. I could picture Lil coming here if she needed to get away from school. Eight-year-old Rosie was so thrilled to meet cousin Lil that she talked non-stop and constantly followed her around. They shared Rosie's room for the night and Lil cheered up a little, being around her.

On Tuesday morning, we left Melinda's for the Carolina Inn, a charming small hotel on the campus. When she was a student, Cate had occasionally been taken there for tea by a wealthy friend, but she never imagined being able to come back with her own daughter. With its classic Southern architecture with large columns and spacious porches, old portraits on the walls and fresh flowers everywhere, it was the perfect backdrop for launching Lil into the world of UNC.

We had a meeting scheduled that afternoon with the head of the disability services, Jim Kessler. Since we were on campus, we were able to walk there, just like students. As we strolled in the warm, summer afternoon, a stream of memories and stories flowed out of Cate.

"Do you smell the magnolias, Lil?" she said as she handed her a big cream-colored blossom.

"That's the bell tower where people used to go to smoke marijuana at "high" noon."

"Don't go in those gardens after dark—perverts hang out there."

When we got closer, Cate realized she didn't know where the disabilities office was. "So much has changed," she said. We ended up in the lobby of the medical school and had to call Jim's office. "Just stay where you are," he told us. "I'll send an intern to get you."

She came and guided us through the labyrinths of the hospital complex to the disability services building.

Jim greeted us and led the way into his office, clearly happy that Lil had chosen to be a freshman at UNC. He had met Cate and Lil the year before when they first toured the campus and he was one of the reasons that Lil was so excited about Carolina. She felt comfortable that they would give her the help she needed.

"If we do our job well, you shouldn't ever need to see me," he had told her.

As we sat in his office, he talked about the things they could do to help her. "Buy your textbooks at the bookstore and then bring them here. We'll cut them up and scan them into files your computer can read," he said.

Then he asked, "Did you get my emails about your room?"

"I don't really do email. My text reader doesn't work on it." Lil looked down, clearly embarrassed to admit that she had ignored his messages.

He paused for a long moment and looked at her while she shifted in her chair, sitting on her hands. "Hmmm," he said. "We'll have to get that fixed."

Then he told her that he had changed her room assignment so that her dorm was more centrally located and she wouldn't have to cross as many large roads to get to classes. It was also a bigger room with space to set up her technology like the CCD camera for magnifying pages and pictures. But it meant that she would room with a senior, not another freshman.

Cate and I looked at each other. From her expression, I could tell we were thinking the same thing: is this a good idea? But Jim must have thought it was. Not wanting to always be critical or complaining, I decided to trust his judgment and say nothing.

Finally, he made her promise to call after Lil got her schedule so he could walk the campus with her to help her get oriented. This turned out to be important, as she was assigned three classes in a row that met in buildings that were far apart. But he had the power to override the registration system and change her class, a great power indeed. It was very reassuring to know that someone on campus could help with issues like this, that she wouldn't have to handle them alone.

That night, in our room at the Carolina Inn, Lil asked me to look over the course scheduling information with her. The meeting with Jim had made her realize she couldn't put it off anymore, that the future had arrived. We spent an hour after dinner going over the distribution requirements and talking about possible courses that she could take.

Because we were there for orientation, they let us move into Lil's dorm room before the rest of the returning students. We hadn't brought much with us in our small car, so we drove to the stores outside of Chapel Hill to buy things for her room. The shelves were packed with back-to-college items, anticipating the arriving hordes of students. We spent the whole morning picking out things to make her room more comfortable and, for the first time, she seemed happy about the idea of setting up her own living space.

We dragged all our purchases back to Lil's dorm room, a big rectangular space perfectly symmetrical on both sides with two beds, two desks, two dressers and a large window at the end. Lil chose the left side. We put her bed up on stilts so that she could fit her desk under it as a former student had told us to do. This made the bed pretty rickety when Lil climbed into it, but she assured me she would get used to it. Cate had found a funky chair in a second-hand store and bought some quilts to cover it, turning it into a cozy little place where Lil could study.

Orientation was held the next morning at the student union. We were the last group for the summer, the out-of-state students, the ones who couldn't come earlier. We started out in one group, the freshmen sitting awkwardly with their parents and eyeing each other, so close to beginning their college life. After a short, forgettable welcome lecture, they took the students off separately and had presentations for the parents alone. Some of these were given in the form of skits by students about what to expect from the freshman year. The presentations seemed to be designed primarily for families who didn't have much experience with going to college, since the message of them all was the same: we had to let go now that our students were at college.

Enough already, I thought. I didn't need this heavy-handed warning to not freak out every time something went wrong. I was familiar with helicopter parenting, having my own experience with advising freshmen. The previous year, a mother had even called me demanding to know why her son was taking a course pass-fail.

"It's required pass-fail," I explained. "Everyone has to take it that way"

"But he's doing so well," she said.

"Then you should be happy," I said without much empathy.

The most enjoyable talk was from the Dean of freshman. He gave a hilarious monologue about how different things were for these students than when he started college. Like a stand-up comic, he talked about how his father drove up to the dorm and just dropped him off, saying, "Call your mother" as he drove away. He contrasted this with the amount of attention students got now. He wanted to make sure we didn't miss the point: "When these kids were learning to ride a bicycle, you ran behind with your hands around them. But now, you have to let us be those hands."

I thought about that talk many times while standing by Lil's bed in the hospital. Such an easy sentiment, such empty words. Where were those hands when Lil was getting sick?

After orientation ended, we asked Lil one more time: "Are you sure you don't want to come to Saltzmann's for dinner?" Marvin Saltzmann was Cate's favorite painting professor and she was excited to get to see him again.

"No, I'd rather stay and get my room fixed up some more," she said, so we dropped her back at her dorm on the way to dinner. I had never met Saltzmann and only knew him from the stories Cate told me, especially the ones where he had devastated students with his withering critiques. I was a little nervous about meeting him, but either he had mellowed with age, or his fondness for Cate made him act kindly to me.

Saltzmann's daughter, Leslie, was also there. We had known her for years, from the time we lived in Albuquerque and Lil was just a baby. When Leslie first graduated from college, Saltzmann had let Cate know she was teaching computer classes that brought her to Albuquerque. We were glad to have her stay with us whenever she came to town. Now she had teenagers of her own.

They both expressed their excitement about Lil being at UNC. Knowing about her eyes, they assured us they would do anything we needed to help—give her rides, take her to the airport, bring her shopping. Saltzmann said he knew some other freshmen and would have them out for dinner when the semester started. Leslie worked on campus in the provost's office and told us to have Lil call her if she needed any help. She promised to take Lil out to lunch after classes started and she wanted to introduce Lil to her daughter, a high-school senior, to talk about college applications.

We left Saltzmann's house glowing from the liquor and good company. Cate had known it would be like this, but I was happy that there were two more volunteers for the network of people Lil could turn to if she needed help. As we got in the car, we called Lil to ask if she wanted us to pick her up.

"No," she said. "I have my cane and I want to practice getting around."

Although she had some training, she hadn't used her cane much before this. Up until now, she had always had us or her friends to drive her around. It was a straight shot from her dorm to the Carolina Inn and she was ready to learn to be independent.

When we got back to the room, we found Lil sitting on the bed, crying.

"What happened?" I asked as we rushed to her side. Cate sat down next to her and held her while she sobbed.

"I was walking back to the Inn and I couldn't find it," she said. Coming from her dorm, she had approached from a different side and been expecting to see a parking lot that wasn't there. She had walked right past the dimly lit Carolina Inn sign on the street.

"I knew it didn't feel right, but I didn't know what to do, so I kept walking. There was a house with a bunch of guys on the porch drinking beer. They saw me with my cane and they started making fun of me."

We had been telling her that people would be glad to help her if they saw her using her cane. Now she said that it made her feel like a victim.

Cate said, "I'm calling the campus police."

"Don't," Lil said, but Cate was already dialing, and was soon telling a public-safety officer what had happened. "Is this the way we can expect our daughter to be treated?" Cate asked. "What can you do about it?"

Cate nodded at the officer's assurances that it wasn't acceptable. Then she turned to Lil and said, "They want to know where it was and they'll go over and talk to them."

"No," Lil said. "I don't want them to. I don't want to be known as 'that blind girl' who got them in trouble."

Cate talked over our options with the officer some more and said we would get back to them if Lil changed her mind.

"How did you finally get back here?" I asked.

"I used my phone. I typed in Carolina Inn and the maps told me where to walk."

I thanked God again that we had gotten that phone. Cate called Melinda and put her on speakerphone so we could listen.

"It must have been one of the fraternities," Cate was telling her.

Melinda started asking for more specifics, trying to figure out which one. She'd been a journalist and her investigative instincts were kicking in.

As they talked, they were getting more riled up. "God, I wish I had a gun," Melinda said. "I'd go shoot out their windows."

As Lil listened to them talk, the fury in these two women made her feel better. She hadn't realized what powerful forces there were behind her, backing her up—the strength of Southern womanhood, family ties and Carolina loyalty.

"What has happened to this campus? How can people act like that? Did you call the police?" Melinda asked.

"Lil doesn't want to let them know who it was," Cate explained and Melinda said, "Let me talk to her."

"Tell me where it happened," she said to Lil. "I'll find out their names and call their mothers. If they found out, those boys would be sorry."

The process of saying goodbye was spread out over a number of days. Lil had to go to one more day of orientation to get registered for classes, but Cate and I skipped out on the parents' part (maybe not setting the best example). The dorms were still empty, so Lil spent one more night at the Carolina Inn with us, cozily wrapping herself in the big down comforter and luxuriating for the last time in the big soft bed. I had to fly back for a meeting in Rhode Island, so Cate took me to the airport early Saturday morning. I kissed Lil goodbye before I left and told her to go back to sleep, as I'd see her again in a few days when I flew back so I could drive the car home with Cate. Cate stayed around Chapel Hill another day to help Lil some more and then went to visit her mother on the coast.

We saw Lil again on Thursday morning before we left to drive back to Rhode Island. Just two years earlier, Lil had been with us when we left Hannah for her first year of college. Hannah had been crying and we were having a hard time leaving. Lil walked up to her, put her hands around her face and looked her in the eye.

"You can do this," she said, patiently, fixing her eyes on Hannah's. She and Hannah often joked that Lil was like the older sister, even though Hannah actually was. Hannah had nodded her head and wiped back her tears. Now Hannah had gone to Montana for her junior year and it was just Cate and me there to say goodbye.

We waited for Lil on the steps to her dorm on a warm, bright, end-of-summer morning. When she came around the corner, she looked like a perfect Carolina co-ed: sunglasses, shorts, flip-flops and a backpack. Her big smile said everything: she belonged here.

She asked us to do one final errand with her before we left, a trip to the bookstore to get her textbooks. It would have been hard for her to do alone, finding all the books on the shelf and getting them back to her dorm. She could have asked for help from the staff, but I was glad we could do one more thing for her before we left.

After a short lunch, we walked her back to her dorm and said our goodbyes in the parking lot. I held her a long time, resting my cheek on top of her head, breathing in the smell of her hair.

"Go," she said. "Don't make me cry."

"What's wrong with that?" I said, sobbing myself.

"Just go," Lil repeated.

She turned away and we got into the car. She waved us off as we drove away. It was hard, but we felt like we had done our best to get her settled. There was nothing left for us to do. The rest was all up to her.

Chapter 22

Tuesday evening, 12/8 -- This morning they did a tracheostomy to put your breathing tube through a hole in your throat instead of your mouth. This was done to make you more comfortable and lessen damage to your vocal chords, because the tube has been in your throat for over two weeks.

The day was pretty quiet and your numbers were okay but not great. At the end of the day, they cleaned you up, changed the sheets and redid the dressings and your numbers went up. Your sats were now at around 90 and we're all hoping it is a real improvement. Cate is very optimistic and starts telling people about how well you are doing. I'm more cautious because the volume numbers still haven't increased.

Lil's coloring was looking good. In fact, she hadn't looked sick or flu-like since the second week in the hospital. The swelling from the ECMO machine was also gone. Since they had done the tracheostomy, she no longer had a tube in her mouth and we could look at her beautiful face. I thought I could I even see a slight smile on her lips. She looked like she was just lying there, resting comfortably. We kept expecting her to wake up any moment.

Chuck left for the airport around 4 p.m., planning to come back on Friday.

I talked to him after he got home and he said that the flight had had a lot of turbulence. Then he told me that it was the same day that his father had died in a plane crash 45 years earlier, when Chuck was only seven. The plane crashed because it was hit by lightning, in the same place that Chuck was flying, just outside of Baltimore. He told me that, while the plane bounced around, he thought to himself, "I can't die! I just did a really nice thing for the Chasons."

Wednesday morning, 12/9 – Your numbers stayed pretty good overnight. The oxygen sats were in the high 80s when I called the ICU at 7 a.m.. Dr. Charles was examining you when I got to your room. Your white blood cell count is over 30,000, which is a sign of infection. This is worrisome, though not unexpected, since you have been on the ECMO so long.

Dr. Charles was concerned that the infection could get out of control. So far, only Lil's lungs had been affected by her illness, not her other organs, but a bacterial infection could change all that. The infectious-disease doctors added some new antibiotics as well as an antifungal agent. She was already getting a lot of antibiotics, but in hospitals they have resistant bacterial strains that are difficult to stop.

Her blood pressure was also dropping. Two weeks earlier, when she had episodes of very high blood pressure, the nurses had told us it was nothing to worry about, particularly in an 18-year-old. Low blood pressure is a bigger concern, as it could be a sign of sepsis setting in. Around noon, her blood pressure had dropped down to 60/40 and they called Dr. Charles to come in.

The last X-ray showed excess fluid on her right lung (the opposite side from where he had put in the chest tube the previous day) so he decided to put in another one on that side. When the nurse told us it was okay to return to the room, he was smiling. He pointed out the new tube that led to a bag full of pink liquid. This is what they had removed from her chest, and now the blood pressure monitor read 140/80. The fluid had been putting pressure on her heart, which was why her pressure had been so bad. Her oxygen level came back up to 86, where it had been in the morning.

Dr. Charles also switched her back to the ventilator they used for burn patients. She was losing air due to a tear in her lungs (like a leaky tire, he explained). This type of ventilator used less pressure, so it would give the hole a chance to heal. Unfortunately, it didn't show the tidal volumes on the display the way the other one had, which meant that the numbers that I had been watching obsessively were no longer available. I wouldn't be able to see if her lungs were getting less stiff and starting to expand.

9 AM Thursday, 12/10 – Cate came in around 4:30 a.m.. You'd had a quiet night, but your sedatives and paralytic drugs were not working well anymore. She said that it seemed like you were trying to talk to her, forming your lips into words that she couldn't understand. It made her feel close to you until you started struggling, lifting your shoulders as you tried to force breaths into your stiff lungs. She couldn't stand to watch, knowing how scary it must be for you.

Around 6:30 a.m., Cate called and told us to come in right away. She had taken the car, the shuttle wasn't running yet and a cab couldn't come for half an hour, so Hannah and I ran the two miles to the hospital.

I told Cate we would get there as soon as we could, then woke Hannah and told her we had to go. We threw on our clothes and ran out of the Ronald Macdonald house and down to US 15/501, crossing it immediately with no traffic at this hour. The long grass alongside the edge of the highway soaked my pants as I struggled to push myself along as fast as I could. I used to be a jogger, but I'd long ago switched to the exercise machines that took less of a toll on my knees. Hannah, a former cross-country runner, held herself back to stay with me. The road to the hospital wound through the campus, climbing at a constant incline that I'd barely noticed when we drove there every morning.

I was out of breath when we got to the lobby of the hospital. We flashed our ID at the security guard and he waved us past. We ran up the stairs and down several long corridors before we got to the ICU. I had to stop outside the door for a moment to catch my breath before we buzzed the receptionist to let us in.

When we finally got to Lil's room, Cate was crying. She was pointing at Lil, who was lying stiffly in the bed, rolling her shoulders, trying to breathe. Cate was begging the nurse to do something. She was already pushing more drugs into the IV lines, trying to increase her sedation, but Lil wasn't responding. The pharmacist had been called but he hadn't arrived yet.

A few minutes after we arrived, the nurse asked us to leave. The nurses had always been so good about letting us be by Lil's side, but this was hard on her, too. Hannah and I held Cate by the arms and told her it would be more helpful if we waited outside. She let us lead her out of the ICU reluctantly, then we went to the lobby and tried to regroup. I said we had to keep in mind that she wasn't sicker. She probably wouldn't recall how uncomfortable she was at times like this.

But Cate couldn't be consoled. It was the first time that she had felt like Lil was suffering and it was tearing her heart out. How long could she go on like this?

We returned later that morning, after they had gotten the sedation back under control. A doctor from infectious disease came over, as she had been doing regularly. They still had no diagnosis, but the white blood cell count was not rising. The broad- spectrum antibiotics seemed to be controlling the infection for now. The new paralytic drug also seemed to be working and Lil seemed to be comfortable again.

Dr. Charles came by later in the morning and asked me if I had seen the X-ray yet. When I said no, he pulled it up and pointed out small signs of improvement in her lungs, little dark spots showing some opening of the lungs. It was the most positive sign we had seen.

1:15 p.m., Thursday, 12/10 – I came back around 11:30 and your sats had increased to the high 80s/low 90s. This is very exciting because it correlates with the improvement in the X-rays. Dr. Charles came in and he seemed very happy. We asked him about what comes next and he laughed and said, "We've thrown away the book when it comes to Lillian." He is clearly more interested in your case than he could be typically. But you have always had that special way of affecting people.

Lil's oxygen sats continued to increase and stayed in the upper 90s, even reaching 100 at some points. Dr. Charles came back that afternoon and conferred with Gary, the ECMO technician. They both seemed pretty excited, so I went over to ask what was going on.

Gary explained that they were going to try turning off the ECMO machine briefly. If her lungs were really improving, then she would be able to maintain her oxygen levels for a while without the machine's help.

Before they started, the level on the oxygen monitor read 98. With a nod from Dr. Charles, Gary turned down the knob on the ECMO machine. I stared at the monitor as Dr. Charles set his watch to keep track of the time. The level dropped slowly. After one minute, it was down to 96. After two minutes it was down to 95. It took more than eight minutes for the level to drop below 90. At that point, Dr. Charles told Gary to turn the knob back to its original level and the value on the monitor recovered to 99.

I could tell how significant this was by looking at their reaction. Neither of them could hide their joy. Gary's mouth was hanging wide open and Dr. Charles was shaking his head, laughing. Dr. Charles folded his arms and tried to maintain his dignity. He suggested waiting awhile and trying again. After 20 minutes, they repeated the test. Again, it took eight minutes for the level to fall below 90 and it recovered back into the high 90s.

After dinner, I put a post on Facebook. I was always hesitant to be too hopeful because of how desperate people were to hear good news, but this was the first time that I felt it was okay to show some optimism. I said her X-rays looked better and ended with, "This is the most encouraging thing we have seen in several weeks. "

The web site had almost 8,000 members now, and messages of encouragement kept coming back all night:

Lillian, you are going to get through this....lilacs are blooming, bubbles are popping and we all love you...

December 10, 2009 at 11:00pm

Way to go Lillian- Tomorrow those numbers will go even higher. Sweet Dreams and rest well tonight.

December 10, 2009 at 10:58pm

It was so wonderful to hear some good news today, Lil. My thoughts are with you and your family. Keep fighting. You're amazing. ♥

December 10, 2009 at 10:46pm

Happy news today Lillian! As you breathe easier, so will we all....

December 10, 2009 at 10:44pm

So excited to hear there is improvement Liilian. You are a true champion, keep on fighting, dont give up. Love and prayers to and your family. Look forward to tomorrow for more great news. :)

December 10, 2009 at 10:43pm

Lil..may you have a peaceful healing night with clearer lungs and higher oxygen saturation levels in the forecast for tomorrow.

December 10, 2009 at 10:43pm

I stayed in Lil's room late into the evening, after everyone else had left. The rest of the world had stopped for me. There was nothing else I needed to do or worry about. Friends had moved in to take care of the house and dogs. My colleagues were kindly covering the end of my class. All I had to do, and all I wanted to do, was be in that room with my daughter.

While the nurse and ECMO technician went about their routines, I stood by the bed and held Lil's right hand, talking to her about the things I was thankful we had done, things that we could have put off or waited until later to do.

I was glad that we had let her have a great summer instead of pressuring her to prepare for college.

I was glad that we had let her get a tattoo, even though at the time I didn't like the idea. Cate had taken her to get it on her 18th birthday and they created the design together—an eye with a heart attached to it—on her wrist, along the heart meridian.

I was glad that we had taken her to Paris during her junior year, so she could see it before her eyes got worse. My favorite picture from that trip was one of Lil twirling around a lamppost on the banks of the Seine, with Notre Dame in the background. My favorite memory came from our visit to the Louvre. When we got to the Mona Lisa, Lil couldn't see it from behind the rope that held back the crowd. With my poor French, I tried to explain to the guard that Lil had a visual impairment. Amazingly, he understood and let her walk past the rope so she could stand eyeball-to-eyeball with the painting.

And I was especially glad that she chose to do what she loved, acting, instead of worrying about whether she'd be able to keep doing it in the future.

3 p.m., Friday, 12/11 – It's hard to believe that it has been three weeks since you entered the hospital. Yesterday afternoon was very good but today has not been as good. Your sats stayed up until early this morning but then dropped, probably after they moved you to take an X-ray. You don't tolerate any movement or changes well, and I don't think the X-ray technicians are always as careful as they could be. Unlike the great nurses, they don't seem to see you as a person and just lift you up like an object when they slide the plate under you.

The latest X-ray showed that the canula were very close together. Dr. Charles repositioned them but your sats only rebounded to the mid 80s. They dropped again after your lungs were suctioned around 8 a.m.

All day, Lil's numbers were lower than they had been the day before. She still had an infection. Her white blood cell count had dropped slightly in the past few days, but now it was back up to 31,000. The source of the infection was probably in all the lines leading into her body. Large bacterial colonies can get established there that are able to fend off the effects of the antibiotics.

The infectious-disease doctors suggested changing all the lines and that made Dr. Charles laugh. It would be impossible to change the canula leading into her neck; she would die during the time she would be off ECMO while they did this. He could change some of the other lines, but preferred not to risk it. He was hoping that she would progress off ECMO in the next five or six days so that we could get rid of the source of infection completely.

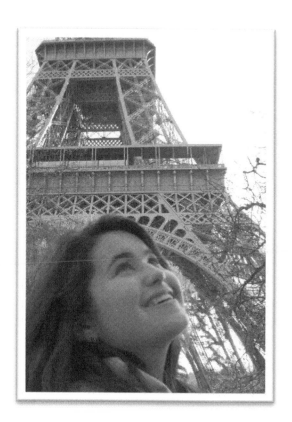

In Paris, April 2008

Chapter 23

The last time I saw Lil before she got sick was at the fall parent's weekend. After Cate and I moved her into the dorm, we decided that one of us should come back for it. Six weeks seemed like a good amount of time to see how she was adjusting. Cate let me go by myself, as she wanted to come down later in the semester so that she could also visit her mother and aunt.

I brought some work and my computer, figuring that Lil might be too busy to spend a lot of time with me. That's how I would have been when my parents came to visit me during college. Luckily, Lil wasn't like me.

I flew down on Friday afternoon and drove a rental car to her dorm. After calling to let her know I was there, I waited on the steps of the front entryway. It was a beautiful sunny day, still summer-like, compared to Rhode Island, with flowers blooming around the walkway. A volleyball net was set up on the lawn between the old stone dormitories. Grills were being brought out for a barbecue that night, and music was coming from an upstairs window. *What a great place to go to school,* I thought.

The students barely gave me a glance as they walked past me into the building. When I first became a professor, I used to think maybe they thought I was one of them. But now, there was no possibility of that mistake. I was clearly one of the parental class.

Lil walked around the corner, the picture of a Carolina girl—shorts and flip-flops, sunglasses, hair pulled back and a big smile on her face. I hugged her hard and wouldn't let go. Her head came up to my chin, and I savored the smell of her hair as I held her.

We went back to her room so she could change. It was the first time I'd seen it since we moved her in back in August. A large pile of clothes filled the big comfy chair. Cosmetics covered her dresser. I didn't realize how much I had missed the familiar scent of them. Her bed was at eye-level, hiked up on the supports that raised it six feet above the ground. It was unmade, the pink and green sheets hanging over the side—new sheets, rather than the familiar ones she had used at home. Rocco Boston, the small, stuffed dog I'd once brought back from a trip to Boston, sat next to her pillow. Underneath the bed, books were open on the desk next to her computer, alongside the CCD camera she used for magnifying her schoolwork.

Her roommate's side of the room was neat and orderly. Lil had told me they got along okay, but weren't great friends. Hardworking and ambitious, she was Chinese and had only been in the US for a few years. She was pre-med and spent all of her time studying. Plus, she was a senior and worried about applying to med school. It was, of course, unusual for a freshman to room with a senior, but the disabilities office had arranged it this way. Seniors got bigger rooms and Lil needed the extra space to be able to set up her visual-aid equipment. The location was also better, so she wouldn't have to cross as many streets to get to classes.

"I don't think she gets me," Lil said. "When I'm lying in my bed, listening to my recorded books, she thinks I'm just goofing off. And she thinks I'm not too smart because I'm studying theater. The other day, she even made some comments about how many sunglasses I have."

I smiled. Lil had a great collection of sunglasses. Oakley's, Raybans, Maui Jim's, other names I'd never heard of. Each had its own case—leopard-skin, silver lamé, camouflage, plaid and leather. It had started when she got her Stargardt's diagnosis. The only suggestion I could find on websites was to avoid too much sunlight and always wear sunglasses. After that, we could never pass a Sunglass Hut without stopping in. Pretty small compensation for losing her vision.

After she changed, we rushed off to see a friend play in a jazz band. As we walked along the path to the music center, she took my arm so I could guide her. She didn't say anything, but it was clear she needed more help seeing than she had before.

At Caribou Coffee after the show, we sat at a table outside, Lil with her legs tucked up underneath her, leaning in to talk to me. Her hands flew around as she spoke, her face animated and lovely. She talked about her friends and what she was doing, her acting and her classes. It was like she was glowing from deep inside.

Meanwhile, she kept texting to make plans for dinner. We ended up deciding to meet her best friend, whose parents were also there for the weekend, and went to a soul-food kitchen where I ate what I wouldn't have eaten if Cate were there.

When dinner was over, we walked back to the car.

"What do you want to do now?" she asked.

"How about a movie?" I said, knowing it was one of her favorite things to do.

"Yesss!" she replied. It didn't let out until midnight, but it was worth it. She dozed in the car as I drove back to her dorm, giving me a sleepy kiss when I dropped her off. "Good night, I'll see you tomorrow."

The next morning I took her to do some shopping. She was excited because she didn't get off campus much, though she had a regular date with Melinda to take her to the drug store. We got some clothes and a refrigerator for her room. That night, we saw a play that she had auditioned for but didn't get a part in and ended with late-night pizza at her favorite hangout. She even got up early on Sunday morning to go out to breakfast before I had to catch my plane. The weekend flew by, but it was pure joy being with her. I hadn't seen her so happy in a long time.

 Cate made her own trip to see her only two weeks before she got sick. Lil's life was busier now, as she'd started rehearsals for the play and had more schoolwork.

"I might not have time to spend with you," she warned Cate. This hurt, but it didn't surprise her. Lil had often kept her at arm's length in the past few years. Better to back off than to insist. Besides, Cate had other family and friends she wanted to visit while she was there.

After checking into the Carolina Inn, she went to meet Lil at her dorm. Climbing into the car, Lil asked if they could go shopping. She hadn't brought her winter clothes down with her and she said she was cold all the time. Cate was happy to take her, as shopping was something they always did well together. But though they hunted through the whole mall, they only found a few odds and ends. Cate picked out a cashmere shawl in a deep burgundy color and wrapped it around Lil's shoulders.

Lil smiled at the warmth of having it around her, but objected when Cate said she would buy it for her, saying it was too expensive.

Cate smiled and said she was glad to be able to do it.

They stopped at the café at Nordstrom's to get a bite to eat before Cate had to take her back for rehearsal. Over their salads, Lil spoke more openly than she had for a long time. UNC was "perfect" and she couldn't imagine a better place. The kinds of things that bothered her in high school just didn't seem so important now. She was still finding the right group of friends. Sometimes, she went to parties and felt trapped. She couldn't leave early and go home on her own because of how hard it was to get around. But she was realizing that she didn't always have to join them, that she liked to spend time by herself. It was okay to want to stay home some Saturday nights and watch TV shows on her computer. And she loved the cast of the play she was working on.

As they drove back to school, Lil talked about her troubles registering for the next semester. Cate agreed, saying it had been like that even when she was a student.

"I can't wait to see the look on my instructor's face when I show up for horseback riding with my cane! It's the only Phys Ed class I could get into."

Then Lil surprised her.

"Would it be okay with you if I double major?" she asked. "It just won't take that long to finish all the theater requirements."

Only a few months earlier, she had said she didn't even want to go to college. And now she seemed so confident. She wanted to do a fine arts major, just like Cate had done, but in ceramics, not painting. She'd taken ceramics during high school and had a real talent for it. Cate treasured the tea set Lil had made her for Mother's Day that year.

"The only problem is I have to take a life drawing class," Lil said.

When she was younger, Lil had loved to draw with pencils and crayons. I had a picture of Billie Holiday she'd made for a high-school class, caricature-like with a huge smile, mouth surrounding the microphone, looking like she might swallow it. It shouted out the joy of performing.

Cate nodded, understanding how impossible that would be now. She suggested that Lil call Cate's old painting professor Saltzman for advice and Lil agreed that was a good idea.

After rehearsal was over, Lil called to say goodnight. "I wish I could spend the night over there," she said. But she had homework to do and needed to go back to her room.

On Friday, while Lil was in class, Cate had lunch with Leslie, Saltzmann's daughter. Since they had reconnected at dinner in

August, they often talked on the phone about Lil and about Leslie's daughter. After lunch, Cate took Lil and several of her friends shopping for food, stocking Lil up with enough snacks to keep going until Thanksgiving. Then they said goodbye in front of her dorm.

It wasn't enough time, but as she disappeared into the building, Cate felt okay about letting her go. This was the best time together they'd had for a while and she felt comfortable that Lil was doing well. It was enough to have accomplished for this trip.

Cate had made plans to visit with family for the rest of the weekend. She drove off to spend the night with her cousin Melinda in their old farmhouse in the country outside of Durham. The next morning, she left to pick up her mother, Tootsie, and bring her back to her Aunt Marky's house in Raleigh. Marky was Tootsie's sister, Melinda's mother and Cate's favorite aunt. Cate was planning to make a big dinner there since she wasn't going to be back for Thanksgiving.

There was no cell phone reception at Melinda's house, so she couldn't check her messages until she was in the car driving away. There was one from Lil.

"Do you think I could come to Marky's with you?" she asked.

Surprised and delighted, Cate called her right back.

"I'm driving there now," she said. "I'll come by and get you on the way."

When she got to the dorm, Lil was waiting, holding the big satchel-like overnight bag Cate had given her. Cate honked and leaned across the seat, pushing open the door for her.

As Lil climbed into the car, Cate said, "Do you want to stop at Marshall's?" That's what they did when we came to North Carolina every summer to go to the beach. We would spend the night at Marky's and the girls would go shopping at Marshall's.

"Really?" Lil said, looking at her in amazement.

"Yeah, Tootsie can wait. This is more important."

This time, their luck was much better, like finding a good fishing hole. Every rack they checked out, they got a bite. Long sleeve T-shirts and pajamas, sweaters and pants, everything Lil needed. They filled up two shopping carts of things to try on. After leaving the store with a huge haul, they stopped and got the groceries for dinner.

They ran into Marky's kitchen laughing, their arms overflowing with bags. Lil stayed at the house to work on her homework while Marky drove with Cate to pick up Tootsie. When they returned, Cate flew into overdrive and prepared a huge feast. Pork roast, asparagus, sweet potatoes. When they served it all up, Marky's husband Bob beamed, "Just like Thanksgiving."

After dinner, Cate collapsed into the big pillows on the sofa, just as she'd done so many times when she visited Marky. Through the windows of the den she could see the stand of pine trees, with cardinals and other songbirds flitting around the bird feeders. To Cate, this house was a magic land, a secret refuge that was always comfortable, welcoming. When she was in college, she had stayed there sometimes when Bob and Marky were away, looking after her younger cousins. When our kids were young, it was the first place we came to from the airport when we visited North Carolina. Marky had made us countless meals over the years, but now she and Bob were getting older. Cate was glad she could return some of the care they had always shown her.

Lil was on the other end of the sofa, sleepily reclining after the big meal they'd just finished.

"That was sooooo good," she said, her hands on her stomach. "I miss good food so much."

"Why don't you give us a fashion show?" Cate suggested.

Lil sprang up and went upstairs to try on and model for them each item she and Cate had found. She reveled in the exclamations of the older woman each time she came down. "Look at how adorable you are."

Cate lay there feeling exhausted but content. This was exactly the kind of thing she'd been looking forward to when Lil chose to go to UNC. They spent the night sleeping side-by-side in her cousin Stephen's room, where Lil and Hannah used to sleep when we visited.

On Sunday morning, Cate drove her back to Chapel Hill and said goodbye again in the dorm parking lot, even more certain that Lil was doing well.

When I picked Cate up in Providence, she overflowed with stories about all the things they had squeezed in and how well Lil was doing. The next morning, she got a text from Lil with a picture. Taken in front of the mirror, the message read: "Picture from Lil in her new outfit" and she had a huge smile on her face.

A few days later, Cate got a phone message from Saltzmann:

"I had a conversation with the lovely Miss Lillian. She told me she wanted to do a major in ceramics. I called the chairman and told him, 'I worked for this department for 30 years. I have never asked for a favor before. But this girl will get a fine arts degree and she will not have to take life drawing'."

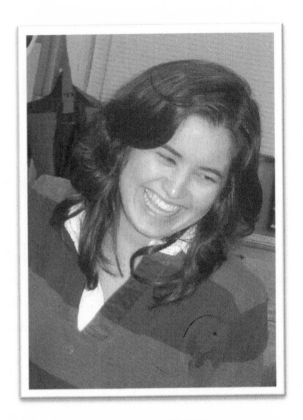

At UNC, Fall 2009

Chapter 24

Friday, 12/11 – It's around 3:45 and I'm taking a break. I haven't had any lunch and I'm feeling sort of low. It's hard when your progress slows down because I want you to get better so badly. It has been a constant roller coaster of emotion, with every up followed by a down. Kathy Short points out that you keep making baby steps in the right direction, but I never realized how hard it is to hope for so long.

Your chest tubes haven't been bleeding anymore and the X-ray from this morning didn't show much change from the day before. The right lung definitely has some open volume, but the left lung shows very little improvement.

It was the first night of Chanukkah. Usually this was a happy night when we lit the candles in the menorah, exchanged presents and ate potato pancakes. I'm not very religious, but this was one of the few Jewish traditions that we observed as a family. The other was Passover. I knew how to run the seder meal because when I was growing up, I went to my orthodox uncle's home for Passover every year. Though at our seders, there were often more non-Jews than Jews at the table. I was also bar mitzvahed when I was 13, which pretty much rounds out my qualifications to practice Judaism.

For Cate's part, I don't think she had even met a Jew until she was in college, there not being a large Jewish population in her hometown of Washington, NC. But she was glad for me to carry out any traditions that I wished. Her father had been among the troops that liberated the concentration camps at the end of WWII, so she had been brought up with nothing but good feelings about Jews. He never talked to her about what he had seen, but it gave him a lot of compassion. The first time I visited Cate's family we arrived, on a Friday evening, and knowing that I was Jewish, he thought I would need to have some kosher wine. The stores didn't carry any, so he bought some NY State wine instead, figuring that was close enough. I don't know what God thinks, but I was pretty touched by it and we always got along great.

Cate is very spiritual but she doesn't follow any organized religion (though she'd been brought up going to a Protestant church). She wanted the girls to have a sense of religious identity, so when we lived in Albuquerque, we joined a Unitarian church. The experience was new to me and I enjoyed the services, especially the singing and the sharing of concerns, the thoughtful sermons and the commitment to social causes. It was hard to object to the open-mindedness of their creed, which someone explained to me in what he called the Unitarian prayer: "Dear God (if there is one), bless my soul (if I have one)." I could accept this, and Cate said that I could be Jew-nitarian.

Attending these services didn't cause any major conflicts in me, unlike the first time we put up a Christmas tree. In my mind, this was not something that Jews did, even Jews as non-observant as me. But Cate wanted one. Her parents had always made Christmas a magical time and she wanted to do that for our children. I did it ambivalently for the first two years, pretending to enjoy it but dragging my feet. Cate finally put her foot down. Either enjoy it, or stay out of the way and she would do Christmas for the girls all by herself.

I couldn't stand being left out of this, so I learned to embrace Christmas. It was all new to me and I loved watching how excited the girls got, waking up Christmas morning and running down the stairs. They were wide-eyed with wonder as they took in the scene of overflowing stockings and piles of presents, some from us and some from Santa.

The one family tradition that we kept from my side of Christmas was going out for Chinese food. Chinese restaurants were the only ones open on Christmas Day, so after the presents were opened and the living room cleaned up, we would head out for wonton soup and egg foo young. Fortune cookies were as much a part of my Christmas tradition as stockings and mistletoe were for Cate.

When we moved from Albuquerque to Providence, we tried to continue going to the Unitarian Church but it wasn't the same. When you're as weakly invested in religious traditions as I am, it's easy to find better things to do on Sunday morning and we slowly found ourselves trading the NY Times for our times with the Unitarians. Cate was starting to search around for alternatives when, not surprisingly, Lillian determined the next stage of our religious life.

When Lil was eight, we attended a Passover Seder at the home of some friends. Passover has always been one of my favorite holidays, telling the story of Moses and the end of slavery for the Jewish people. Our hosts also had a mixed marriage and two boys who were younger than our girls. The husband's father had been a rabbi, so he knew what he was talking about. He asked the kids lots of questions and told lots of stories. Lil was mesmerized.

On the way home, she said "Next year I want to read the four questions."

Cate looked over at me with a look that said, "Your turn" and asked what we had to do to be Jewish. The girls waited for an answer from me, the expert in the family.

"Usually you do it by being born to Jewish parents."

"Well, duh," said Lil.

"I'm not converting," Cate added quickly.

I thought about it for a moment more as I drove, wondering where this was going to lead.

"I went to religious school when I was your age. To get ready for my bar mitzvah."

Lil said, "Then that's what I want to do."

Cate was fine with the idea of the girls being Jewish, even if she didn't want to convert herself. She just wanted them to have some religious practice. After calling some Jewish friends, she confirmed that the synagogue in Barrington was a good match for what we wanted. We joined the congregation and Cate got Lil registered for religious education. Hannah didn't want to be left out so she asked if she could go, too. Lil was starting early enough to be ready for her bat mitzvah at 13, but the rabbi said Hannah would have to go just as long and wouldn't be ready until her 16th birthday.

For the next few years, we car-pooled them to Hebrew school for two afternoons every week and Sunday school on the weekend. We had to start preparing for the bat mitzvahs more than a year before the actual date—find a place to have it, get a caterer, music, and a million other things. We gathered the girls to talk about it.

Lil was excited. "Won't it be cool?" she said. "My birthday is in March and Hannah's is in April. We'll have two Bat Mitzvahs in two months!"

We hadn't discussed this with them before but two separate ceremonies made no sense. We couldn't ask people to come twice, and we certainly couldn't afford to do it twice. They would have to do it together, we explained. At first they didn't like the idea, but they got used to it pretty quickly. The novelty of sharing it and splitting up the ceremony helped.

The day of their B'nai Mitzvot (the term for two ceremonies) was a beautiful day in May. Aunts, uncles and cousins who I hadn't seen for years came from all over. When I was young, we all lived in the New York area and we got together a lot. But since then, our family had become pretty spread out geographically and we didn't see each other often. The girls didn't know many of them and were amazed to learn that they had so much family on my side.

Cate didn't know them well, either. The only time she had met many of them was 18 years earlier. We had been living in Tokyo where I had taken a one-year post-doctoral research position after finishing my Ph.D. I went there in September and Cate joined me the following February, after she finished writing the thesis for her Master's degree. Her joining me was an acknowledgement that we were committed to each other and that we would get married. Because her family and mine lived so far apart, we decided to get married in Tokyo in May. Then we would have wedding celebrations when we returned, one in North Carolina with Cate's family and another in New York with mine.

A few weeks before we returned home, my father told us he would need another by-pass operation, as the one that had been done 10 years earlier was beginning to fail. I asked him if he wanted to wait until we got home, but he said he wanted to get it over with.

The night of the operation, we waited by the phone (it was late night for us with a 14-hour time difference) and couldn't understand why my mother didn't call. Eventually, the phone rang.

"They can't get his heart started again," was how she explained it. The doctors said they were still trying, but there wasn't much hope. She called back an hour later to say he was gone.

It was a complete shock. My mind just couldn't accept it. My only coherent thought was that I needed to get home. My mother was by herself, unlike the first time when we had all been there to wait together—my brother and his wife, my sister, me. But this time we thought it was routine, he'd already been through it once. I told her I would be there as soon as I could.

We were supposed to leave in just a week, so we had already started preparing. I fumbled around, trying to think of all the things I needed to do, never having experienced anything like this before. I phoned my boss and explained that I had to leave. Cate was going to stay to pack up and join me later.

As I was starting to call the airlines, she asked whether I wanted her to come with me. I still wasn't used to thinking like a married couple. We'd lived together for several years but had only been married for a few months.

But when she said it, I realized that I didn't have to do this alone, that I had someone to share this with. Packing wasn't important. So what if we just left everything behind?

When I called my boss again to tell him Cate was coming with me, he said not to worry. He would get our apartment packed up and have everything sent to us (when the big shipping boxes arrived six weeks later, even the garbage we had left in the apartment was neatly wrapped). He picked us up early the next morning and drove us to Narita airport. Luckily, the Japanese like to do things with cash, so I was able to withdraw all the money we had earned from the ATM machine at the airport. It spit out a whole year of savings in a large stack of 10,000-yen notes that I brought over to the American Express counter and converted into traveller's checks.

The flight home took 28 hours, with an overnight stop in Toronto. Cate slept some, but I mostly sat in stunned silence, thinking about my father, still not able to believe he was gone. We flew into La Guardia and my aunt and her son picked us up. The terrible sadness in her face over the death of her brother made it a lot more real. We drove for an hour to my family's house in the suburbs. In the Jewish tradition, people come to the house of the deceased person so that his family is not alone. Ours was packed. Cate had never met most of them and it was a strange mix of feelings. People expressed their condolences one moment and their congratulations on our marriage the next.

Cate and I were travel-ugly and exhausted. After a short time, she excused herself and crashed in my old bedroom. I was tired, but floating on adrenaline, so I stayed up late into the night talking to my brother and sister. Out of these reminiscences the three of us prepared a eulogy that we delivered at the funeral the next morning.

After the funeral, Cate and I stayed with my mother for a few days while she figured out what to do next. We eventually returned to our old apartment in Cambridge while I worked for one more year at Harvard and looked for a permanent job.

With my father gone, we didn't feel like having a wedding celebration with my family in New York and we called it off. So the funeral was the one time Cate had met many of the people who were now arriving for the B'nai Mitzvot. It was a lot better this time to be meeting for a joyous occasion, and many people observed that my father would have loved it.

Marky and Bob escorted Cate's mother Tootsie to Rhode Island and I was grateful to them for accompanying her. Bob is a very religious Christian man and I first imagined that he might be uncomfortable at a Jewish ceremony but I was completely wrong. He was fascinated by it and peppered the rabbi with questions afterwards. Confident in his own faith, he was eager to learn how it fit in with his understanding of the Old Testament.

All day, I just couldn't stop smiling, greeting all the people who had travelled so far to celebrate this milestone with my family. And the girls were absolutely perfect. Poised and beautiful, reading their parts of the Torah, sharing the ceremony with each other, graciously thanking the many people who had helped them get this far. We held the reception at the Brown faculty club and it felt just right, neither too fancy nor too plain. It was one of the happiest days of my life.

Lil didn't continue much longer with religious school after that. Earlier she had been curious to learn about the Jewish traditions, but now she was turned off by the rigidity of the rabbi. She had lots of questions and instead of feeding her curiosity, he tried to tell her how she should think. I picked her up one afternoon and she recounted her latest exchange with him.

"I don't believe any of this," she said she'd told him. "I didn't write it, you didn't write it, so why do you have the authority to tell me what to believe?" This made her a hero to the other kids in the class, but didn't curry favor with the rabbi.

Another time they'd been discussing the Holocaust.

"The rabbi told me that I wouldn't have spoken up," she said. "That I would have just done what they told me. But I told him that wasn't true. He doesn't know me."

I had seen Lil stand up for the underdog before. One time on the playground, she had stopped others from bullying a child with learning disabilities. Just like her mother, she had a strong moral compass and wasn't afraid to stand up for what she believed. I don't know what anyone would do in a situation like Nazi Germany, but what was the point of telling her she wouldn't resist? It was clear that she had reached the limits of what she could get from this form of religious education.

But she still liked to think about the big questions. She argued with a boy who tried to tell her that losing her eyesight was God's will. On her Facebook page she had written that her religion was: "When I do something good, I feel good. When I do something bad I feel bad."

When I was visiting her at UNC, she told me that her favorite class was Religion and Philosophy. Here the professor didn't mind being asked tough questions, discussing the different arguments for God's existence. If God was all-powerful, then why was there suffering? But if God wasn't all-powerful, then how could he be God?

The class was held in the evening and there were many adults in it who were taking it through the continuing education program. An older gentleman had recently stopped Lil after class to say he enjoyed her "delightfully cynical" perspective. She was proud of this. Why should she accept the other people's view that this must be a perfect world because God is watching over us? She told me her experience with her eyesight gave her the right to question things that others didn't.

My own ambivalence about religion didn't stop me from being thankful whenever anyone said they were praying for Lil. It was really all that anyone could do. Many churches put prayers for Lillian in their Sunday services and many prayer groups included her, as we learned from letters and entries on Facebook. When her teacher, Mark Perry, posted that he wanted to have a prayer meeting at the hospital, hospital security came and asked us to have him call it off. They were worried that they couldn't handle the number of people who would come.

The collection of religious artifacts on the shelf behind her bed continued to grow: vials of holy water, a candle with the image of our Lady of Guadalupe. Ribbons holding prayers to saints were added to the collection of objects hung from the IV pole. Every time Cate went back there to add something to it, it made me nervous because she had to snake between a complicated tangle of wires and tubes. Recently, she had started allowing the nurses to do it after one of them told her about accidentally knocking out a hose and blood spraying all over the room.

Leslie had stopped by after work with an electric menorah for us. After the sun went down, we asked the nurse, Patrick, to put it on the window sill with the other religious objects. Patrick was a large man, well over six feet tall, but he moved calmly and gracefully around the hoses and cables hanging from the racks and jutting out from the wall. He plugged the menorah in and twisted the first light in the highest socket so it shone like a candle.

Hannah and I recited the Hebrew prayer out of habit, feeling strange to be saying it without Lil's voice joining in. For years, the girls would fight over who got to light the first candle. Hannah explained to Patrick that the one next to it needed to be lit also, because the center one, the "shamas," was used to light all the others.

The next morning. I saw the poem that Cate had written on Facebook:

A steady joy
Pushes out from Lillian's small half window.
A slow stream of hope emanating from this dense building,
This house of miracles.

Patrick methodically moves through end-of-shift motions.
His large mass, a graceful dance around her bed.
Hovering over IV lines,
Replacing one of a dozen bags --
Plastic orbs hanging from five poles.

A liquid show of gravity
Forces slow drips of carefully discussed,
Meticulously calculated pharmaceuticals.
Into Lillian.

His 6'5" to her 5'2"
Two and one half times her density --
Carefully he swabs her eyes and lips with moisturizer.

Patrick, a mass of humanity
Who graciously nurtured
My baby through this first night of hannukah
A healer who comes back,
Shift after shift.

If need be,

He could easily
Lift her in his arms
And cradle her like an infant,
Like a new life come to us.

Like the way the new moon holds the old moon in its arms.

Chapter 25

Saturday, 11:55 a.m., 12/12 – Chuck came back last night with his wife Kathie. Your blood pressure went up as we talked by your bedside. It seems that you get agitated when you hear us—probably due to the difficulty of keeping your sedation at the right level. They have told us it is difficult to sedate teenagers because their metabolism just eats it right up.

In the past, your blood pressure spiked several times during the night but now it seems to be a little better controlled. I woke up at 4 a.m. and called the NSICU. The nurse said your sats stayed up in the 90s. It is so exciting that you didn't have any setbacks last night.

Dr. Charles repositions your chest tube so he can remove fluid from your lungs. More than a liter of fluid comes out. The blood in it is deep red (new blood would be a brighter red) so hopefully there isn't new bleeding. He replaced the tube with a larger one so that it wouldn't clog up as easily. Your sats are still good after the procedure. Now we're waiting for the results from another X-ray to see whether the lungs show any improvement after removing all that fluid. There are still many complications to watch out for, including your infection.

Chuck and Kathie came over to the ICU in the mid-morning. Cate had gotten there before dawn, as usual, and Hannah and I arrived on the first shuttle after breakfast. Kathie produced a large bag of her famous oatmeal cookies that Cate accepted eagerly. She loved having the goodies that people sent us to distribute to the nurses.

Kathie was a very special person to Lil. She had been her mentor for her senior project, allowing Lil to shadow her in her work as a speech therapist with kids who had severe developmental disabilities. Kathie was amazed by how unfazed Lil was by their problems. One boy just wanted to hug her and she allowed him to, sitting still without being uncomfortable. When she came home, Lil said that she could imagine working with kids with disabilities if her eyesight kept her from being able to be an actress.

Dr. Charles came in and was happy to see Chuck again. The latest X-ray didn't show any improvement. The left lung still wasn't opening up. The doctors discussed it and Dr. Charles thought that there was a clot in the space between the membranes surrounding the lungs (the interpleural space) where the fluid was collecting. The chest tubes should have removed it, but not much was coming out. He asked us to leave so that he could reposition the tube. After moving it he was able to remove over a liter of fluid.

The progress she'd made in the last few days meant that we wouldn't have to talk about terminating ECMO on Monday (as we had discussed at the meeting the previous Monday). As Dr. Charles had said, Thursday was "perfect." We just hoped that her sats would get to be as good again as they had been then.

Lil had been in the hospital for three weeks and people were anxious to see her. We hadn't wanted to have lots of visitors and told most people to wait until she got better. But when Thom and Charise asked if they could come, we couldn't say no. Thom was the one who'd come over with his partner, Kevin, to help with Lil's college applications. He was like one of the family. Lil joked that she couldn't decide if he was more like a brother or an uncle so she called him a "bruncle." Tall and handsome, he had been an actor before becoming a voice coach and they had a very special bond. He had helped her with her singing, but it was more than that. We'd had countless meals together, and Lil was always excited whenever he came over. Sitting on the couch before dinner, she would curl up next to him like a puppy. And Thom adored her back, laughing with his big voice at the comments she would make during dinner.

Lil and Charise had gotten to know each other when Charise was a grad student studying drama at Trinity Rep in Providence. She stayed with Lil for several days when Cate and I went away during Lil's senior year in high school. Since then, they had stayed in touch and gotten very close, like sisters.

"Where have you been all my life?" was how Charise described it. She had finished school the year before and was living in New York trying to get work as an actress, travelling a little further up the career path that Lil was hoping to follow. They talked all the time and Lil had even gone up to NYC to visit Charise during her fall weekend break.

Thom flew down from Providence and Charise from New York City and they met at the airport so they could come together to the hospital. A nurse came in to tell us when they got to the locked door of the ICU and Cate went to escort them in. I met them as they walked around the curtains that defined Lil's room. We all exchanged hugs and greetings as they took off their coats and scarves, asking them things like, "How was your trip?" and "What time did you leave?"

When they saw Lil, Thom reflexively bowed his head and folded his hands in front of him, as if he had entered a church. Charise took his arm and they stood looking at her in silence, tears forming in Thom's eyes.

I was so used to the routine of the ICU that it was easy to forget how it must appear to someone coming in from the outside world. I filled them in on her status, and Cate told them where they could stand so they could talk to her while being careful not to disturb the IV lines and wires.

Thom went up to her first and talked for a while in a hushed voice, holding her little hand cupped between his large palms. Then he gave Charise a turn.

She had lost her mother to cancer a few years earlier so she was unfortunately familiar with the hospital atmosphere. You could see that sadness in her body as she sat on the edge of the bed, whispering into Lil's ear.

We stayed around Lil's room talking for a while, giving them a chance to be with her. But we had been there all morning without eating and we needed to get some lunch. At first, I told the others to go without me. I didn't want to be too far away if anything went wrong. But Chuck suggested that I could call the ICU from the restaurant to make sure everything was all right, so I agreed to go.

It was a beautiful afternoon and we decided to walk to the Mediterranean Deli, one of Lil's favorite restaurants in Chapel Hill. We each went to a different counter and ordered large plates of food — Greek salad, grape leaves, lentils and rice — then brought them back to the table to share.

It felt good to get away from the hospital. I called the ICU after we had eaten and they said nothing had changed, so I felt okay about having left..

The long walk back gave me a chance to talk with Charise. I wanted to hear about Lil's visit to see her a few weeks earlier. I had known a lot about the trip because I'd helped Lil work out the logistics. It was going to be the first time she had ever flown by herself and we talked about what she would need to do. She almost cancelled several times, saying she had too much work or it was too hard, but I encouraged her to go.

This time, when people saw her using her cane, they were helpful, unlike when she got lost in Chapel Hill. At the airport in North Carolina, the people at security helped her find her gate and the agent there told her where to sit and when to get on the plane. When she arrived in New York, a transit cop helped her get a taxi, and waited until she got in. She handed the driver a slip of paper with the address that she had written out beforehand and he took her straight to

Charise's door. This was very fortunate because, unknown to me until then, her neighborhood in Brooklyn wasn't particularly safe.

That night, they stayed up way too late, talking and laughing, drinking coffee, sharing stories. They were both night owls and now there was nothing to make them stop. They each understood about loss and weren't afraid to talk about it, sharing their difficulties about getting adjusted to the new places where they were living.

Charise talked about how hard it was to find someone to have a relationship with and they went on a dating site to try to find a boyfriend for her. They looked at the pictures and read the descriptions of potential suitors, laughing at the transparently false bio's, yet finding a few who seemed promising.

Lil talked about her troubles getting around campus and they looked at sites for seeing-eye dogs to see what Lil needed to do to get one.

They slept late and went out for brunch the next morning. Walking through Prospect Park, they marveled at the beautiful color in the trees. Lil put a photo of herself on Facebook that showed her standing under a huge yellow tree, the sun and the leaves creating a glow around her. Her arms were open like she was catching the leaves, her face smiling as if to say, "Isn't this glorious?"

The focal point of her trip was going to see a production of *Our Town* (which was one of my favorite plays). I always thought that Lil would be perfect for the role of Emily, the young woman at the center of the play. "Do any human beings ever realize life while they live it— every, every minute?" Emily asks.

Lil had that same beautiful innocence and honesty in her own soul. In one of her high school roles, she played the girlfriend of a boy who became an addict, and her pleas to give up drugs and come back to her had the teenage boys in the audience crying.

Charise told me how the play was staged, with the actors coming into the audience to interact with the people watching it. The character of the stage manager took special notice of them, coming back many times. It had been like he was talking directly to them:

"We all know that *something* is eternal. And it ain't houses and it ain't names, and it ain't earth, and it ain't even the stars—everybody knows in their bones that *something* is eternal, and that something has to do with human beings. .... Aren't they waitin' for the eternal part in them to come out—clear?"

"Lil and I held hands for two hours and we cried," Charise told me. "We stayed in the theater for a long time after it was over. Then we took the train back to Brooklyn. Lil dropped her head onto my shoulder, and she just kept on crying."

She said that Lil asked her again and again, "Am I appreciating it all enough?

"Why do I worry so much about my homework and my play and my friends when life is so short? Am I taking things one moment at a time? Am I too obsessed with getting it all right all of the time?'

"I kissed her head," Charise told me. "I said to her, 'Lil, no one appreciates life like you do. No one can see like you do'."

I had my arm around Charise's shoulder now. She was small, about the same size as Lil, and it felt like it was her that I was walking with. As we went past the Carolina Inn. Charise put her arm around my waist and leaned her head against my chest, just like Lil would.

"You know she really loves you," Charise said. "She talked about you a lot. She often said, 'My Dad says this or my Dad says that ...'."

I couldn't stop the tears from streaming down my face as we walked the rest of the way back to the hospital.

We spent the rest of the afternoon in and around the ICU. Having all of us in the room at the same time was a lot, and we didn't want to get in the way of the nurses and technicians, so we took turns going out for walks and coffee. Nobody felt like eating dinner after the big meal we'd had. Cate left around 7 so she could get to bed early. Thom and Charise left around the same time because she had to catch an early flight back to New York. Kathie went back to the Inn and Chuck stayed with Hannah and me into the late evening so we could make sure Lil was stable.

Her blood pressure still kept spiking periodically, the numbers on the monitor rising suddenly like her body was slamming the accelerator to the floor. The alarm on the monitor went off and the nurse (it was Patrick again) calmly walked over to it and turned it off.

The stillness of her body was hard to accept. The monitors were telling me that her heart was going at a rate higher than I could ever get to by exercising, yet she lay there peacefully. Patrick increased her sedation but he didn't want to do it too quickly or he would have to use other drugs to reverse it. It was agonizing to wait and see whether her body would respond or whether he would have to give her more. I could feel my own heart racing, panic creeping over me as my heartbeat pounded in my ears.

I wondered what effect all this sedation was having on Lil. They checked her eye reflexes regularly and her pupils were normal size and showed a "brisk" response to shining a bright light in them. The nurses told me that people can wake up from this type of medically-induced coma after a long period and show no cognitive impairment, so I was hopeful that she would be able to recover fully when her lungs got better.

Her muscle mass had also decreased significantly due to the combined effect of the paralytic agent and the steroids. She had been in great shape before getting sick, but now her arms and legs were stick-thin. Dr. Charles told us that she would go back into the pediatric ICU when she got off ECMO, which made us happy. The nurses there really loved her—they had kept coming to the NSICU to check on her progress ever since she'd left their unit. Then we would probably go back to RI to continue her rehab.

I liked to imagine Lil being in a rehab facility near our home and thought of all the friends who would want to exercise with her and help her recover her strength. I thought of how much fun it would be to lie with her and watch movies together like we always loved to do. It was getting nearer to Christmas and I was sure she would want to catch up on all her favorites: "Elf," "Love Actually," "White Christmas," even if we missed the holiday season.

Sunday, 12/13 – Last night you were pretty stable but your sats were down a little, in the high 80s and low 90s. I spoke to the nurse (Patrick) at 4 a.m. and he said your blood pressure still kept spiking periodically. Each time it does, they respond with more sedation and have been able to get it back to normal.

On Sunday morning, Thom took Charise to the airport before the sun rose for her early flight back to New York. Then he surprised Cate by coming back to join her at the hospital in her early-morning vigil. She told me later that they sat by Lil's bedside and talked for a long time and she could tell that Lil knew he was there. Cate described her as being "all lit up." After Thom had to leave to catch his own flight, Cate said it was like the light went out.

When I came in around 8:30, the first thing I did was look at the monitors, as always. After they'd stabilized Lil's blood pressure last night, it hadn't gotten out of control again and the oxygen sats were around 89. This was not good and not bad, so I wasn't expecting any major news.

But the nurse was excited when she called me over to the computer to show me the latest lab results. They sent blood off to be measured around every 6 to 8 hours and these results were a much better indicator than the numbers that we watched on the screen in her room.

I saw a screen full of numbers and wasn't sure what she wanted me to notice. She told me to look at the color, and I said I didn't see any, the numbers all appeared to be black.

"That's the point," she said, delighted. "They've all been red up until now because they've been outside the normal range. But these are within normal."

Later that morning, Dr. Charles came in and checked the latest X-ray on the computer. It was nominally better and he decided to reposition the chest tube on her right side to remove more fluid (just as he had done with the left side earlier). That went well and she remained stable all afternoon.

When the sun went down, we added another light bulb to the menorah. Now there were three bulbs lit, along with the center one—five more left to light through the end of the holiday. We could see them glowing every time we went out to make phone calls in the passageway on the other side of the hospital that overlooked her room.

Sunday evening, 12/13 – Dr. Charles came in to check on how you are doing. We talked for a while and when he left, he said that he was going home. It had been a bad day. Chuck walked out with him and they talked briefly. When Chuck came back, he told me that Dr. Charles had lost a patient today who they were trying to put on ECMO. He had been working on her all day, ever since he had repositioned your chest tube. But they weren't able to get her blood flows to stabilize and she died. I think that he came in to see you just to feel a little better.

Chapter 26

The week after Cate visited her at UNC, Lil got more and more busy. As the end of the semester approached, lots of assignments were coming due: watching a six-hour performance of "Nicholas Nickleby," preparing a presentation for drama class, writing another paper for religion.

She also had rehearsals every night for her play. Up until this point, she'd been able to stay on top of her work, but it was beginning to pile up. She was trying not to panic. Just like her last two years of high school, it was stressful, but she could handle it. She'd just work extra hard. And there was only one more week until she could go home for Thanksgiving break.

On Saturday, she stayed in her room to work on one of the papers. It was a sunny autumn day and the campus was alive with people streaming in for the last home football game of the season. Her friends kept texting her to join them but she stuck to her plan to get some work done. She finished her paper in the late afternoon, took a shower and walked over to the stadium at halftime. It felt good to have made a dent in her workload and now she could enjoy taking a break. After texting back and forth, she finally located her friends in the crowded stands, next to the band. Later, she hung out with another friend, Dillon, whose brother was visiting and listened to them play guitars in his dorm room.

The next day, she woke up with a headache. *Damn*, she thought, *I can't afford to get sick, now.* As the day wore on, it got worse and turned into a stabbing pain behind her eyes, unlike anything she had felt before. Around noon, she texted us to ask for the number of the eye doctor at Chapel Hill.

Cate was in the yard raking leaves and I was working on my lectures when we got the message. Cate called and gave her the number of the retinologist; she had already registered Lil as a patient in the beginning of the semester. She told her to drink plenty of water and get some rest.

Cate spoke to her later that afternoon and again on Monday morning. Lil was worried about missing classes but Cate reassured her it was more important to see the doctor. She wasn't able to get an appointment until 8 on Tuesday morning. In the meantime, her eyes hurt so much that she was afraid she was losing her remaining vision. In all the time since her diagnosis of Stargardt's, Cate had never heard Lil so worried.

After they were done talking, Cate immediately called the disabilities office. She wanted to speak to the director who knew Lil, but he wasn't there. She spoke to an aide who often helped Lil and arranged for them to take her to the eye doctor the following morning.

Cate wrote to Lil on Tuesday morning before the appointment: "You will feel better soon. You are an inspiration."

After seeing the doctor, Lil was relieved to report that the problem was not her eyes. He told her that she probably had a virus and she should go to the health services. Too tired to go from one appointment to the other, all she wanted to do was to go to her room to rest. Cate made her promise to go the first thing next morning.

When Cate called back an hour later, Lil said she couldn't breathe well.

"I could call Leslie or Melinda to take you to the health services," Cate said, but Lil told her that she was too tired to get out of bed.

"I could come down to help," Cate offered but Lil was emphatic.

"No. Other kids have it. I'll be okay."

Cate had to force herself not to call again so that Lil could sleep. After what seemed like an eternity, she texted her late in the afternoon:

> Curious to know how you are feeling. Talked with Leslie. She said she would call you every day until you feel better! I wish I could be there for you. Torture all around. Love you

Lil called back an hour later and said that she still couldn't breathe well and she would go to the infirmary the next morning.

On Wednesday morning, Cate called Leslie and asked if she could take Lil to the doctor. When they got to the health services, the waiting room was packed. The H1N1 flu was raging and the staff was overwhelmed. The university's main concern was limiting the spread of the disease. Parents had received emails earlier in the semester about what students should do in the event of the flu. If students lived nearby, it was suggested that they go home. If not, they were encouraged to get a "flu buddy," somebody who could bring them food and liquids. They were told to keep to themselves and limit contact with others.

Lil slumped into a chair, her head pounding, all of her muscles tired, all of her effort going into trying to breathe. The receptionist wanted to send Lil back to her dorm but Leslie explained that she wasn't just feeling bad, she couldn't breathe.

The triage nurse sitting in the room behind them leaned out of the door and told the receptionist that Lil needed to see a doctor. They couldn't get her in until 1 that afternoon and the doctor would be double-booked, but they would make sure she was seen.

Out of Lil's earshot, Leslie explained that Lil also had a vision problem and they needed to make sure they got her back to her dorm. Then Leslie had to leave and Lil continued to wait by herself.

The nurse escorted Lil into an examination room and took her vital signs. Her heart rate was 112 per minute and she had a fever of 100.7. Her chest felt tight and she told the nurse about the trouble she was having with breathing.

The nurse gave Lil a machine to blow into to measure the peak flow of her lungs. The first time she tried, it measured 250. At Lil's age and size, it should have been over 420. She was in great shape, having rowed all summer and taking advantage of the exercise classes in the gym. She had never had breathing problems—no asthma, no allergies.

The nurse wrote the number down and told her to do it again. This time she made it up to 300.

"One more time, Honey," the nurse said. "This time try real hard."

Lil mustered all her strength and blew once more, getting the meter up to 350, the minimum acceptable value. The nurse put the numbers in Lil's chart with the annotation "poor effort."

The nurse gave Lil some Tylenol before the doctor came in to examine her. He listened to her lungs and they sounded clear to him. Her neck wasn't stiff and her fever was down slightly. But she was clearly having trouble breathing and her heart was racing.

"Any wheezing?" he asked.

Lil shook her head no. She probably seemed scared, breathing fast and shallow. If he asked, she probably told him she was worried about her classwork. Maybe he thought she was just a panicky freshman, away from home, over-reacting to a little sickness. She may not have looked him in the eye since she couldn't see his face.

He wrote in her chart: "Reassurance given with normal vitals and exam. Recommend rest and copious fluids. I expect her to develop new symptoms (nasal, cough, etc.) over next few days."

But there was no diagnosis. No explanation for why a healthy 18-year-old should be short of breath. No request for a chest X-ray to look at her lungs.

"You can take Aleve for the pain," he told her. "But don't come back for a few days. You're going to be fine."

Then he sent her back to her dorm.

Why didn't he send her to the infirmary, you might wonder? Because there isn't one. Like many universities, UNC doesn't have any place to send sick students except the hospital.

Did they do any follow up? Did anyone call to check up on her? Was there any system to monitor students who were sick? Even ones with disabilities?

We were in the middle of a nationwide epidemic. The Centers for Disease Control said students should promptly seek medical attention if they developed severe symptoms, including shortness of breath. It was well-known that young and healthy adults were at the greatest risk of getting serious complications.

Yet the institutional plan for a school that housed more than 15,000 young adults was to call your flu buddy and ask them to bring over a drink. Or go home if you were lucky enough to live within driving distance.

But what about an 18-year-old kid from out-of-state who had never lived away from home before? Who always did what she was asked to do. Went to the health services when she was sick, just as she was told. She had severe symptoms, just like the CDC had warned. And the only thing they did for her was to send her back to her room with reassurances.

A disappointed Lil called Cate afterwards to let her know what had happened.

"All he did was tell me to go back to my room. He said I'll probably get worse and I shouldn't come back for a few days."

"I can be there tonight," Cate said. "You've already missed classes. We can fly home together. Or get a hotel room."

"No," Lil said, and threatened to stop calling Cate if she suggested it again.

Cate agreed, but only if Lil promised to let her know how she was.

That night, Leslie stopped by with some chicken soup that Lil gratefully accepted. She was encouraged by the fact that Lil wanted to eat anything. On the way out, Leslie stopped at the RA's office to make sure they knew how sick Lil was. The RA wasn't there, so Leslie left a message with the person on duty, but no one ever came by to check on Lil.

Cate called again that evening to see how she was doing.

Lil told her about the soup and assured her that her friends were bringing her things to drink.

When Cate asked about getting help from her roommate, Lil said she wasn't there. "She volunteers in the emergency room on Wednesdays," Lil told her, without seeing the irony.

After midnight, she texted with Dillon. He had been sick, also, but was starting to get better:

D: Are you sick too? We could have had a sick party.

L: You're sick! Dude I'm dying an bored!

D: Yeah fever and shit. It's starting to go away though. I think. Can't be too sure. What you got?

L: The bubonic plague.

D: Well do you have meds and stuff? I've got some extra tylenol pm if you need it. Shit works wonders.

L: Oooo pm drugs sleep

D: Want some? I'll bring it over real quick

L: Would you really? Because icannot fall asleep

Lil stayed in bed all day Thursday.

Cate texted in the morning but got no reply. She called her at 1 p.m. and Lil said she couldn't breathe unless she was lying down.

Cate begged her to go back to the doctor but Lil insisted she follow his instructions to not come back for at least two days. She was putting on a brave face for Cate, but inside she was feeling alone and scared. She wrote to her friends, asking them to bring her something to drink. Most were busy with their own work or didn't respond, but some got back to her:

L: I really feel like I'm dying

ZMB: Dont worry it has to go away soon. Is there anything you need?

L: I don't know I feel like I can't breathe but yesterday they said it was nothing

Can you grab a bunch of packets of those saltine crackers too. There by the soup. And straws please. I'm sorry.

ZMB: On my way to the dining hall now

L: Thanks buddy

Later that night, Lil tried to call Leslie. She didn't have her home number, so she left a message on her office phone. It said that she was feeling worse. Maybe she would have asked for a ride back to the health services if she had talked to her. But Leslie didn't get the message until the next morning.

In Rhode Island, Cate was going through hell. She desperately wanted to go down to her, but Lil insisted on acting grown up and independent. She wouldn't let her mother come down just because she was sick.

And I was no help at all. I thought I was being reasonable, telling Cate not to worry, that it was only the flu. I hadn't spoken to Lil myself because the one time I'd called, I woke her up from a nap and didn't want to do that again.

So I just assumed that Cate was overreacting. Stupidly, ignorantly, I told her the same thing they told us during orientation. She's growing up, we have to let her go. We have to trust that they would take care of her.

The next morning, Cate called to check in. Lil had gotten up in the middle of the night to use the bathroom and didn't have the energy to climb back in the bed, so she slept on the floor.

"I'm calling Melinda," Cate said, and immediately phoned her cousin. Melinda knew that Cate might need her and was ready to go.

When Melinda got to the dorm, she called from the parking lot to let Lil know she was there. Lil came staggering out of the front door, looking like she was drunk. After helping her into the car, they sped down to the health services.

This time, the doctor immediately recognized the severity of her symptoms. She was quickly taken to the emergency room.

Melinda told us later how brave she remained, calmly answering the doctors' questions as she lay flat on her back, the only position that allowed her to breathe. When they put in an IV to hydrate her, the nurse brought a bedpan, but Lil insisted on getting up to walk to the bathroom. Melinda had held Lil's hand when the doctor explained that she needed to go on a ventilator, and was by her side when they put a phone to her ear so she could talk to us.

"Then she dried her tears," Melinda said. "She asked if I would stay. I said I would, and I gave her a kiss."

Melinda stayed with her all day until after she was admitted to the pediatric intensive care unit. In the evening, she had to leave to take care of her own children.

Leslie was at home preparing a dinner party for her husband's birthday when she found out that Lil was in the hospital. After the party ended, she drove over to the hospital at midnight to sit by Lil's bedside so she wouldn't be alone. She was still there when we arrived the next morning at 5.

Chapter 27

Monday, 12/14 – Last night you were stable but your sats were down a little in the morning. This was a typical pattern. You were doing well when we left for the night, but overnight you had several episodes during which your blood pressure spiked and your sats decreased.

They switched the ventilator back to the conventional one so we were able see the tidal volumes again. Based on your progress over the past few days, we were hoping to see some increase. But the number (around 130 mL) is less than it was on last Monday before they added the new canula and your heart stopped.

This was very disappointing, since you'd had a few good days in a row. We were hoping to see more compliancy in your lungs to go along with the X-rays, which seemed to be showing some clearing up. But the doctors are still expecting you to get better and come off ECMO, so we just have to keep waiting.

That night, Chuck and I sat and talked quietly in her room until about 10. I felt more comfortable if I was near her and he kept me company by her bedside. The numbers on the monitors weren't significantly better than they had been in the morning, but we imagined that they were starting to show improvement, with the tidal volume sometimes flirting with 150 mL.

After returning to the Ronald MacDonald house, I went to the computer room to post something about her status. I looked over the last few updates—so many ups and downs since her heart had stopped a week before:

Update: Wednesday, 8am

"Yesterday was much quieter than Monday (thankfully). Lil was stable all day and then her oxygen saturation rose some in the afternoon (from the low 70s to 90) which is a good thing. It stayed in the high 80s all night which may indicate her lungs are getting ready to start opening up. Her volume still hasn't increased, which has to happen as her useable lung space gets bigger. But it is hopeful sign."

Update: Thursday, 11am

"Yesterday was a long day after the improvements on Tuesday. She has an infection but it seems to be responding to new antibiotics. As Dr. Charles and the nurses remind us, it is two baby steps forward and one step back. She rested through the night and got back to sats of 85, but became uncomfortable this morning at 5 AM when the sedation wore off. It was hard to see her uncomfortable, but it also shows she is still fighting. The pharmacist is working hard to keep ahead of her as she builds up tolerance to the different medications. But she seems to be comfortable again -- now we are waiting for her sats to recover and the healing process to continue."

Update: Thursday, 7pm

"The first thing that Dr. Charles asked this morning was had I seen the X-ray yet. When I said no, he pulled it up and he pointed out the first signs of improvement in Lil's lungs that we have seen. There are now some dark areas that were previously white, showing that the lungs are less fluid-filled in some places. She is on a new type of ventilator so we can no longer measure her tidal volumes (the number that we want to reach 500). But her oxygen saturation has also gone up considerably (into the 90s most of the day). She is still fighting off an infection and there are many other potential pitfalls, but this is the most encouraging thing we have seen in several weeks."

Update: Sat, 8am

"Sorry I wasn't able to post yesterday. It was another long day with lots of ups and downs (but it ended up okay). In the morning her sats were down, especially after they took another X-ray. They remained down, probably because the catheters that bring and take her blood to the ECMO machine have shifted position. Dr. Charles adjusted them several times over the day (it's a minor surgical procedure) and they finally came above 90 in the afternoon. I spoke to the ICU at around 4 AM and she stayed stable throughout the night. Her X-ray yesterday showed slight improvement (definitely no worsening). She still has an infection which is always something to worry about."

Update: Sat, 9:30pm

"Dr. Charles performed a procedure today, replacing one of the tubes in her lungs for a larger one, and a liter of fluid was drained out. This should help her to breathe better. Her blood pressure and pulse and oxygen levels stayed relatively steady. Little by little she is getting better and we try to stay patient."

Update: Sun, 10:30pm

"It's Sunday evening and we just left Lil for the night resting in her room. She's had a good day. Dr. Charles changed the chest tube in her right lung to get out some more fluid. Her sats have been steady throughout the day and the x-ray showed some improvement from yesterday. Her blood pressure still rises rapidly... some times which we take to mean she is becoming more aware. They treat it with additional sedation. She's still in a race to get off ECMO as soon as possible, but every good day helps her heal more."

There were many positive signs: her heart was strong, the infection was limited to her lungs, her color was still good, the infection wasn't getting worse, the X-rays showed positive signs.

But we hadn't yet seen that big change we were looking for, where she turned the corner and her lungs started to expand. We just had to keep believing that it would happen.

I wrote another post summarizing the day's events:

> "Another day of slow progress. They changed her ventilator so they could measure her tidal volumes. They were still small when we came in this morning -- only around 125, similar to the last time. But they slowly crept up to 140 by the time I left her tonight. They still need to get to around 300 to get her off ECMO ...(and for Dr. Charles to dance) so she has a ways to go."
>
> Dec. 14 at 10:37 PM

Tuesday, 12/15 – In the morning the news wasn't good. Your sats had stayed up overnight, but the lab measurements of the blood gas had declined significantly. The oxygen partial pressure went down from 51 in the previous evening to less than 40 over several consecutive measurements. Dr. Charles did a bronchoscopy at 6 a.m. and both Cate and I were there to watch. Your lungs still looked pretty good in the larger air passages that could be seen. There was less redness and there wasn't a lot of blood during the suctioning. He also adjusted your left chest tube, trying to remove fluid around your lungs, but not much came out. The latest X-ray didn't show much improvement.

At 1 that afternoon, Dr. Charles held a meeting to discuss the options in front of us. He gave us another deadline, saying he would discontinue ECMO on day 30 if there wasn't improvement. That would be next Wednesday, still eight days away.

Chuck talked about doing more recruitment of the lungs, in which they increase the pressure of the ventilator to try to force the alveoli open. Since they don't have ECMO in RI, he is used to trying to treat conditions like Lil's with more aggressive ventilator strategies.

But the risk is that this will tear the very stiff lung tissue and lead to bleeding. Dr. Charles listened, but said that he wanted to hold off a little longer. He would consider it if things didn't get better in the next few days.

4 p.m., Tuesday, 12/15 -- You are stable all day and your volume increases to 150 mL so there are some hopeful signs. Your sats are in the high 80s and your blood gas is a little better (around 44 mm Hg).

Chuck and Kathie left around 3:30 but they planned to come back over the weekend. There was a blood drive for Lillian at UNC that day. Her friend Zealan had organized it after we told him about how much blood they needed for the ECMO program. They got 47 units before they ran out of capacity. They sent another 10 people over to a Red Cross drive going on at the same time. We estimated that Lil had used about 70 units, so at least we had made up for some of that. That evening, Zealan brought over a huge card that everyone had signed for her.

The television news was there to cover it, and we watched the report on the computer that evening. More and more people were hearing about Lil and sending their thoughts and prayers. Nine thousand people were signed up for her Facebook page and many more were following. Messages were constantly coming in, urging her to get better.

We had to start seeing some improvement for her to get off ECMO. I stared at the numbers on the monitor, hoping that they would start to rise. I imagined it as if we were in a movie—the numbers would start going up as everybody got more and more excited.

Why wouldn't that scene play out for us? Or maybe it was just getting ready to happen. Whenever there was a slight improvement, I hoped that we would be able to look back at that point a few days later and say, "Oh, see? That's where it was just beginning."

Wednesday morning, 12/16 -- Before Chuck and Kathie left yesterday, your tidal volumes were showing values as high as 150 mL. It looked promising, but later that evening, they started to drop a little. Dr. Charles came in about 6 p.m. and took out more fluid through the chest tube. The subsequent X-ray was better than any we had seen.

I came back after dinner hoping to see some improvement in your tidal volumes, but they remained lower than the day before. The nurses changed your sheets because the chest tube was oozing. As usual, you didn't respond well to the added stimulation. Your ECMO technician wasn't the best we'd had, and she seemed like she was almost falling asleep. But I assumed it would be okay overnight.

By the time that technician's shift ended the next morning, Lil's sats were very bad. The oxygen monitor went down to 47. A new technician came in at 7 and he got it back up to around 90. But the morning X-ray showed more seepage of fluid into Lil's lungs and he told us he was worried.

Cate, Hannah and I wandered in and out of the room all morning, sitting in the chairs and reading magazines, taking breaks to make phone calls, drink coffee or write on the computer.

Around noon, I was in the corridor walking slowly back toward the NSICU after checking my email on the computer in the waiting room. Over the hospital PA system there was an emergency call for the respiratory therapists.

I stood to the side as a number of people ran past me dressed in scrubs. I hadn't really been paying attention until I saw the ECMO technician, Gary, sprint by me and into the NSICU.

I grabbed the NSICU door before it locked and hurried through. From the end of the corridor, I could see that most of them had gone to the room next to ours where there was an elderly patient. When I got to our room, Gary was in there, doubled over, trying to catch his breath while he talked to the ECMO technician who was on duty. The technician was assuring Gary that things were okay, that the call wasn't related to Lil. The patient in the next room died shortly after the emergency was called.

Wednesday afternoon, 12/16 -- They had been trying occasionally to recruit your lungs by raising the peak pressure on the ventilator. To see if this was expanding them, they decided to take an X-ray of your lungs while the pressure was elevated. The X-ray was scheduled for 4 p.m. so the respiratory therapist came in before that to adjust the ventilator. Your sats had dropped again and raising the pressure didn't show any loosening of the lungs.

They shot the X-ray and afterwards, her sats dropped into the 40s again. This time, the technician couldn't get them up again by adjusting the ECMO machine.

Cate called Dr. Charles on his cell phone, but he didn't come right away. She tried calling again but he didn't answer. He arrived shortly afterwards and we could tell by his body language that things weren't good. Normally he was rushing around trying to fix something or find out something, but this time, he was subdued.

"We've been giving her a lot of blood products and it must be going somewhere," he said.

This was a surprise to me. It didn't show up on any of the monitors that I could see, so I didn't know about it. There wasn't any obvious bleeding—her stomach wasn't distended.

He did a bronchoscopy, expecting to find bleeding in her lungs, but they were still pretty clear. When he had finished, he cleaned up and then walked over to us.

We looked at him expectantly, waiting to hear what he would do next.

"I don't think there is any chance for her to recover," he said. "She's been on blood thinner so long that fluid is continually pouring into her body."

Refusing to hear this, we asked him what could be done. "There must be something," we begged.

For the first time he didn't have anything new to suggest. He reminded us that he always said that after 14 days the danger of bleeding from ECMO would rise. They could keep going, but her other organs would start to fail.

"But she was stable just a few hours ago."

He shook his head. All he said was that they could turn off the oxygen supply to the ECMO machine. Without its support, her heartbeat would only continue for a short time and then she would be gone.

For three and a half weeks we had lived on hope. Recovery always seemed to be lurking around the corner. Over and over, we had told ourselves it would be here soon. It was just a matter of time.

"We'll put her on a respirator to help her breathe until her lungs get better. "

"We'll put her on ECMO for a few days. She'll go home just like the H1N1 patient in the bed next to hers.

"If it takes a little longer, well that's what they've been seeing in Australia. It could happen at any time, just like a switch being thrown."

Her heart had stopped, but then she'd come back, a miracle like no one had ever seen. A few days later, her oxygen levels got up into the normal range. If she could just hold on a little longer, give her body a little more time for her lungs to heal. Why wouldn't they just clear up?

Now I was being told that there was no more hope. No future with the little girl I had carried everywhere in the crook of my arm, who threw her arms around my neck as I leaned down to pick her up, who called me Daddy and gave me sleepy goodnight kisses. The baby who loved to press her nose into my nose as we touched foreheads and sang songs to each other.

My beautiful baby would never get to have babies of her own. The beautiful actress who mesmerized audiences would never get to star in her first lead role at UNC. Her performances would only remain in a handful of DVD's, taken with my shaky hand.

Dr. Charles told us that, if we wanted, he could discontinue the sedation so that Lil could be conscious briefly before he stopped the machine.

I looked at Cate and Hannah to see what they thought and the look on their faces mirrored my own feelings. I couldn't imagine anything more cruel than to wake her up only to learn that she was about to die. Even though it would have been priceless to have one more conversation, it would be kinder to keep the sedation on. She'd always seemed to be resting comfortably, so this would allow her to slip away quietly and peacefully.

I asked Dr. Charles to put the ventilator on the maximum settings, just in case her lungs might start to work again on their own, one more final chance.

He did, and then he and the nursing staff and technicians left the room to give us a chance to say goodbye. We had already had several weeks to be with her and tell her how much we loved her. There had been several times when we thought we were going to lose her and had to face the possibility of death.

But now the actual end had come and this was our last time to be with her.

We stood around her bed and took turns saying goodbye. I held her hand and told her how much I loved her. She looked so restful it was hard to believe that these were going to be her last moments of life. I moved around the bed to give Hannah her turn, but I didn't feel like I was in control of my own body. All I felt was numbness and a deep, deep sadness beyond anything I had ever known before.

When we finally told them it was okay, they turned off the oxygen to the ECMO machine. For a brief period her sats stayed up and I hoped that maybe there would be another miracle and her lungs would start to work.

But soon, her blood pressure started dropping, and then her pulse rate decreased. She never struggled or seemed to suffer as we said goodbye.

Then her heart quietly stopped beating.

.   .   .   .   .

It had all seemed to happen so quickly. We had been by her bed for weeks, but things completely turned around in just a few short hours. There had been so many times that she had had reversals before this and then was able to come back. We had always had something to hope for, some progress to look forward to, some monitor to keep our eye on.

But now there was nothing. Nothing to do, nothing to hope for, nothing to look forward to. If I had the power to stop time, it would never have moved forward from there. How could I still breathe, walk, feel, when one of my main reasons for living was gone?

"That would be a waste," I could hear Lil saying. "If I can't be there, that's no reason for you to give up."

It was the only consolation I could find.

We couldn't leave the room. We wanted to talk about Lil, to let everyone know how special she was. They had never gotten to meet her and they had to understand.

Cate told Dr. Cairns that he should see Lil's college essay. She turned on her computer and it was in a mode where it spoke everything that she typed, just like the software that Lil used to read documents out loud. Cate had never used that mode before. We were sure it was a sign from Lil.

The nurses worked quietly and considerately in the background, covering Lil with a white sheet and unhooking her from the equipment. As word spread around the hospital, doctors and nurses silently appeared from other units to give us a hug and tell us how sorry they were. I always knew they cared a lot, but I was still surprised by how much it seemed to affect them. But as much as I could see others crying, it couldn't touch the pain I felt.

The head nurse let us use her office so we could make some calls. We needed to speak to some people directly to let them know. We called friends in Rhode Island and in North Carolina and asked them to go to our mothers' houses so that they wouldn't be alone when we called. Other friends called Matt's parents so they could break the news to him. They immediately got in the car and drove 5 hours up to Maine to bring him home from college. When they arrived, the resident advisor met them and said he had been sitting in his room the whole time, banging his fist on the wall.

We went to the Carolina Inn to spend the night. It was too hard to go back Ronald Macdonald House. Leslie drove us there and asked them to re-open the kitchen so that we could get a bite to eat while she sat with us.

I knew that we had to post something on Facebook because people were beginning to find out about her passing. Someone had already written RIP on her Facebook page (we don't know how they found out) and we immediately removed it. I don't remember writing it, but somehow I posted the following:

"I'm sorry to have to tell everyone that Lillian died this afternoon at 5:20 PM. Her sats kept dropping during the day and Dr. Charles said that the ECMO machine could no longer keep her supported. As you all know, she put up an incredible fight and if there was any way she could have overcome this disease, she would have. We want to say thanks again to the wonderful people at the UNC hospital who have been and remain incredibly supportive. And thank you all for all your prayers and kind thoughts -- it was an incredible comfort during this long difficult journey."

The next morning, Hannah and I went to Lil's dorm room with some friends and UNC staff to pack it up. Cate stayed back at the Carolina Inn. It was too hard for her to face.

After living at the hospital for the last few weeks, it was a shock to be suddenly transported back into Lil's world, surrounded by the objects of her everyday life. Her bed still unmade, her clothes scattered around her side of the room, the make-up sitting next to the magnifying mirror, waiting for her to start the day.

I thought of all the trips we'd made to Target and the second-hand store to find just the right furniture. The cozy chair with an old quilt to snuggle up in, a good floor lamp to help her read, an extra computer table for the CCD camera that let her magnify her books. It was a life that she was enjoying so much, a life that she would never resume.

In her closet, I found her sunglass collection. Each case held its own world of memories, reminding me of when we bought them, and the girl who wore them. When we first found out why she couldn't see the baseball well enough to pitch anymore. The time that Matt, always protective of her, had asked whether it was safe when she took them off to be photographed for her senior prom. We had thought her eyesight was going to be her big challenge in life, and we had no clue as to how blind we could be.

We drove away around 1 p.m.. It was a strange feeling leaving Chapel Hill, since we'd always had such warm feelings for it. We had looked forward to visiting Lil there for years.

We were on the road in Virginia when the phone rang, about the same place where the driver had stopped in the middle of the night when he took us to the hospital in Chapel Hill from Baltimore. It was Melinda, who was helping to make the funeral arrangements by coordinating with the funeral home in Chapel Hill. Dr. Charles had asked us to allow them to do an autopsy, so Lil would remain in Chapel Hill for a few days. But there was a big winter storm coming and the funeral home was concerned that they wouldn't be able to get her to Rhode Island in time.

After Cate hung up, she called Dr. Charles to ask him about the scheduling of the autopsy. She was surprised when his wife, Celeste, answered the phone. She told Cate that he had taken the day off and was still in bed.

Chapter 28

Wednesday, 12/23 -- It's already been a week since you died, but I haven't had a chance to write again until now. Even though I'll no longer be able to tell this story to you (at least not directly), I feel a strong need to finish off the narrative of what has happened. I want to have something that I can share with other people, so they can have some understanding of your remarkable life. A week ago, I wrote:

Thursday, 12/17 -- We got as far as Maryland on Thursday night. It was good to drive back. Cate and Hannah and I were able to be together and the transition didn't have to happen too quickly. It would have been difficult to fly up to Providence and be thrown immediately into a homecoming. You would have understood. You always enjoyed road trips, with the comforting rhythm of being in the car as the miles roll by.

I had posted a brief message on Facebook the night Lil died. The outpouring of shock and grief was immediate and immense. That night, more than 300 people wrote messages of condolence:

> MA: Oh, Eric, Cate, Hannah, I feel like my heart has been ripped out - I can't imagine how you must feel, I just can't imagine. We share your grief. Rest in peace, Lil – you deserve that much, after such a battle.
>
> December 16 at 11:25pm

> CC: Lillian touched and inspired so many people, and I am honored that I was able to work with her. Such a talented and caring girl. Rest in peace, Lillian - you will always be in my prayers and thoughts.
>
> December 16 at 9:36pm

TV: I am so very sorry for your loss. There are no words, but do know how many lives have been touched by hers, and by her brave battle. As a parent, I am so very, very sorry.

December 16 at 9:27pm

BG: Dearest Lillian, It is in your light that we know love. You will shine forever in our hearts. Rest sweet Lil.

December 16 at 9:43pm

SZT: I am honored to have spent the last two years working with your daughter-my heart is breaking for you....she had so much left to give this world......she will be missed.

December 16 at 9:45pm

LHE: My heart is broken. I will never forget you, beautiful Lillian.

December 16 at 9:46pm

Seven hundred more messages were posted on Thursday and Friday. It was amazing how many people wanted to share expressions of regret, remembrance and love. A whole community of people who had never met was grieving for her.

We woke up early in the motel room but took our time getting ready. Even though there was a lot to do, we didn't want to get home too quickly. The drive went smoothly until we got to Connecticut, where we crawled along in traffic for a few hours.

Suddenly, Cate started crying, shouting out the questions we didn't ask while we were hoping for her to get better. "How could they send her back to her dorm all alone? Why didn't they give her Tamiflu? Why wasn't there an infirmary where she could be watched?"

I was driving and Hannah was sitting next to me. We looked at each other as Cate wailed in anguish in the back. There was no reason to argue with her or try to calm her down. All I could do was nod in agreement.

When we got back to Barrington in the evening, we couldn't face going to the house right away. We needed to stay in our bubble a little longer.

Cate's friend, Pat, had been talking to her everyday and was one of Cate's biggest supports. Cate told me to drive to their house first, and they had a glass of wine and a bite to eat for us when we got there. Talking to them gave us a little chance to unwind before facing the reality of being back.

When we finally got to our house, there were flowers and cards on the kitchen table and casseroles in the refrigerator. Nanda, the woman who had been housesitting and watching the dogs for us, was ready to leave as soon as we got there, knowing we needed our privacy.

After letting the dogs settle down, Cate walked upstairs. Hannah and I brought some of the things in from the car, then I went upstairs, too. I walked into Lil's room and Cate was sitting on the bed. A candle was on Lil's dresser and I went over and read the note from a friend who had dropped it off.

Neither of us talked. The pain was too great to try to say anything.

I opened the closet and stood in front of it for a while, staring at the clothes hanging there that reminded me of her, not able to believe that she wasn't coming back.

Saturday, 12/19 – We knew we had a lot to do today: picking out a grave, talking to the chaplains about the service and going to the funeral home. Pat and David picked us up at 10 a.m. and we went to the cemetery first.

We had never had to do anything like this before and appreciated Pat and David being with us. We wanted to find a site at Swan Point, an old cemetery on the east side of Providence. Park-like and beautifully landscaped, it's a place that Cate and I used to go to for walks during lunch. It was alongside the river, near the boathouse, and Lil used to row past it when she practiced.

Pat and David had gone there the day before to pick out the best sites so we wouldn't have to look at too many. Pat had even sent us pictures of some of them from her phone.

We immediately liked the gravesite that they had picked as the best. It faced south and had trees nearby, not too sunny and not too shady. A few plots away was a monument of a beautiful weeping angel.

Afterwards, they took us out for some lunch at a restaurant near the downtown mall. It was packed with people shopping. We'd forgotten that it was less than a week before Christmas.

Next, we met with the chaplains from Brown to arrange the service. They were wonderful at listening to what we thought Lil would have wanted. The chapel at Brown was too small, but the minister of the Unitarian Church told them we could hold the service there, remembering that we used to be members a long time ago.

When we were done, Pat and David picked us up to go to the funeral home. Picking out the casket wasn't as difficult as we had expected. We all agreed on a simple one made of poplar with beautiful wood grain. Melinda had written an obituary that they sent to the newspaper. It captured Lillian's spirit beautifully:

> Lillian was a joy, a talent, a beauty and a force to be reckoned with. She had strong opinions, a fierce intelligence and a sweet heart. She lived her life in all directions, bright and extravagant. She was, and is, a magnificent soul. The

best lives take unpredictable turns; when we least expected it, Lillian soared, and sails under the gale force of the spirit.

The only hitch was that there was a big snowstorm coming. The autopsy had pushed back the schedule and the plane with her body had only gotten as far as Atlanta when the connecting flight was cancelled. I had heard jokes about people being late for their own funeral but I didn't know it could actually happen. In the worst case, we were told we could have an empty closed casket during the visiting hours if her body hadn't arrived. In the face of all we had been through recently, it just didn't seem to be something we needed to worry about.

Sunday, 12/20 – It started snowing around 9 p.m. Saturday night. By Sunday morning, there were 18 inches on the ground. We laid low. Neighbors came over and kindly shoveled our driveway. Julie Wilson came over with some dresses for Cate and Hannah to try on. That evening, the Sherman's came with dinner for us and Pat and David brought some soup.

It was really good for me to see Chuck Sherman, again. I needed to know from him that there really had been hope for Lil's recovery and that it hadn't been futile.

He told me they really believed that she was going to make it. After they left North Carolina on Tuesday, he had talked to Dr. Charles, who had said he thought we might have to meet again the following week if Lil didn't show improvement, but not that she would be gone the next day.

The whole ECMO team was devastated, he'd told Chuck. They were much more invested in her case than any other he had ever seen. Even at the hospital, many people had been following her progress on Facebook and feeling the outpouring of love and support for her.

They had told the staff not to post on it because they didn't want them getting too involved, but it didn't matter. They were going to have a meeting of the whole group on Monday because they realized that the people who did ECMO were going to need more support and counseling than they expected.

By Sunday afternoon, we got a call that said the plane had left Atlanta and would be arriving on Sunday night. We were relieved, but it barely registered; by now we were pretty numb from all the ups and downs that had occurred over the past month.

Monday, 12/21 – Monday morning was clear and bright and not too bitterly cold. We went to the cemetery to finalize the purchase of the grave. Then we went to the Seven Stars Bakery where you had always loved to go. Cate said that the Tibetan Book of the Dead said we should eat the things that you loved to give you comfort. So we split a chocolate almond croissant, one of your favorite things in this world. Pat and David came to our house around 3:15 to take us to the funeral home for the visiting hours. They were scheduled from 4 to 8 p.m and we wanted some time with you ourselves before the crowds arrived.

We had decided to put Lillian in the black dress that she had worn to her senior prom. She had told us that she had never felt more beautiful than she did that night. It was sleeveless so we had them cover her arms and shoulders with the burgundy cashmere shawl that had been around her in the hospital, the one they had bought on Cate's last visit. Her hair was clean and beautiful as always. It was arranged to cover over where her trach tube had been. Her face was lovely, although Hannah remarked that she looked a little pissed off.

I thought it would be hard to look at her, but the sight of her in the casket, with her favorite dress on and all the flowers around her, was actually very beautiful. I knew that she would have been pleased, and that gave me a lot of comfort.

We stood and greeted people for the next five hours, an hour longer than they had allotted. There was a steady stream of people the whole time—the line went out the door and into the parking lot. So many people wanted to say goodbye.

The last person to come to the viewing was our friend Dorothy, who had flown in from Albuquerque. She had been present at Lil's birth, holding Cate's hand, supporting her during contractions, telling her to breathe. So it made sense that she was also the last person to say goodbye at the funeral home.

After the last visitor, the rabbi said some prayers for closing the casket and it was over.

> *Tuesday, 12/22 -- We held your funeral on Tuesday morning on a bright, cold RI morning. Your mother noted that your visitation was held on the shortest day of the year, but your funeral would be on the day that they started to get longer.*
>
> *There was still lots of snow on the ground, but the air felt soft. We formed a small caravan outside our house, led by the limousine from the funeral home, and drove to the Unitarian Church, where the family and closest friends assembled in the back room.*

It was the most lovely funeral I've ever been to and I think Lil would have been happy with it. We had readings by many people who loved her, each speaker bringing alive a different part of her, making me wince and smile at the same time. Sandra Lambert read a poem chosen by Cate and remarked about her amazing ability to get so much done, "like she was running a small country." We sang the hymn, "Morning Has Broken," which Lil loved listening to from Cat Stevens.

Her friends had gotten together to write remembrances and several of them read them aloud. Lil would have been proud of them. It always bugged her the way people would dismiss teenagers from our town as spoiled and uncaring.

Their words went by too quickly, so I asked them later to send me what they had written. Katie Baldwin captured how Lil could switch instantly from serious to non-sensical:

"(you) always provide a piece of wise advice, and sometimes a piece of ridiculous advice you would think was hilarious and then attempt to convince me to actually do it."

Emilie Shore's included this:

"When you laughed, really laughed, I found myself wondering how someone so tiny could produce something so powerful. It seemed as though it came from some outside force. No matter what you were doing, your laugh took control... Tears would stream from your eyes and it was impossible for anyone near you not to be happy."

The hardest part was when Matt spoke. The tears streamed down his face, and his shoulders heaved. I'm not sure how he was able to get out the words:

"... I always felt childish in deep conversations because she just seemed to always understand, and always know herself. I used to think that maybe it's because she questioned everything, never following blindly. Or maybe it was part of her incredible strength, stemming from learning to cope with her eyesight problems."

My favorite part was when he recollected talking to her about losing her vision and he said that if he were in her place, he would focus on music. But she responded that she wouldn't, because "becoming a blind musician was too cliché." That sounded just like her.

I remarked to his mother later how she had always worried that she would break Matt's heart.

"She did," was all she replied.

Annie read one of Cate's poems and then Thom sang "Til There Was You" in his big actor's voice, one of the most beautiful things I had ever heard.

I walked up to the front of the church to say a eulogy. Chuck walked alongside me in case I needed help. Sitting in the pew, I hadn't really looked at the crowd but now I could see it.

The Unitarian Church is a beautiful space in the classic New-England style and it was filled with people, on the floor and in the balcony. The winter light came through the side windows in strong, brilliant beams. Later, someone told me how the sun had moved through the sanctuary during the service, from the back to the front. By the time I spoke, it was shining directly on me and where Cate and Hannah were sitting.

Cate had been worried about me being able to read it, but there were some things that I wanted to make sure people knew. When she was sick, we hadn't talked about Lil's eyesight on the Facebook page and I wanted people to know how bravely she had dealt with it. I tried to summarize other highlights of her too-short but magnificent life, her love of acting, her outspokenness, her tremendous intellect and things that I knew other people probably wouldn't say.

Strangely, it reminded me of their B'nai Mitzvot, the only other time I had gotten to talk about her in public. I was so glad now that I had that chance five years earlier to tell her in front of others how much I loved her and how proud I was of her.

Finally, the rabbi read the mourner's Kaddish, a traditional Jewish prayer, and we listened to a variation on "Simple Gifts," a reminder of the Quaker summer camp she loved, which she had gone to for years.

After the service, we went to the cemetery. I couldn't see how long the line of cars was that followed us, but there were many people at the gravesite. After a prayer, we took turns putting a shovel of dirt on the coffin, another Jewish tradition. The rabbi explained how the shovel is turned upside down while doing this to make it harder, symbolizing the difficulty of saying goodbye.

The light in the cemetery was as amazing as in the church; there was a shaft of sunlight shining directly on her grave during the entire burial.

We got back in the limo and I later heard that Matt fell apart at this point. He threw a rose into the grave and then collapsed into his parents' arms.

Pat and David had arranged to have a reception at the Rhode Island Country Club. The big windows of the clubhouse looked over a snowy field leading down to the bay. One table was filled with all foods that she loved and another table had shots of milk and chocolate chip cookies. Her friends projected a slide show they had made and played a CD of her favorite songs along with it.

We stayed for a long time, and eventually a smaller group went into the bar and continued talking. We finally had to go home to a very empty-feeling house.

Wednesday, 12/23 -- The day dragged on. Friends stopped by the house and out-of-town people came over to say goodbye. That evening, we sat shiva, another Jewish tradition where people come over to our house.

More observant Jews sit shiva for a week, but we were just going to do it for one night. Cate had reminded me how Lil had learned about it in Hebrew school and said, "Now I know what to do if somebody dies."

Kathie Sherman came over and cooked us dinner before the other people arrived, another nice tradition. I was worried that Cate might not like having so many people there and told her she should go upstairs if she wanted to. Instead, she stayed holed up in the kitchen surrounded by the close friends who made her comfortable. When I looked over to find her, she was surrounded by a wall of good, strong woman who I felt would keep away anyone she didn't want to see.

Thursday, 12/24 -- We started off the day slowly, each of us writing and taking our time getting up. Around 10, we went to walk the dogs at Brickyard Pond. Pat came over with an armful of Christmas presents. She didn't want us to not have a Christmas this year. It was very kind, but it hurts to think Christmas will never be the same without you. We've been showered with tons of food and other friends came by to eat and keep us company.

Christmas Day, Friday, 12/25 – So here it is Christmas Day and our worst fears have been realized. We can't comprehend that you won't be here again to share our Christmas, or tell me about your life. It doesn't make any sense and it isn't fair, but I don't think fairness or sense have anything to do with it. It is clear to me that we are always walking a narrow tightrope, not acknowledging how close we are to falling off at any time. Strangely, I had always been conscious of the possibility of loss. You would make fun of me because every holiday, I would always marvel at how lucky we were to be all together and that another year had gone by without a major tragedy. I knew that we were the luckiest people in the world.

As I sat missing her on Christmas morning, an image came to me from the blood drive that they'd held for her. Several people had written that they had wanted to come to UNC to give blood directly to her and didn't know if they could make it in time.

I wrote back to them and said that it doesn't work that way, that they could give wherever they lived and it would go into a pool that all could use. Lil had received blood from people who never knew about her, and the people who contributed would be doing the same thing for someone else.

It occurred to me that maybe love is like that, too. We can't always love the person we want to directly, because they are gone, or aren't able to receive it now.

But maybe love is meant to be shared by all—we should love those around us while we can, and hopefully the love will spread to others who we can't be with.

Lil certainly received love from many people in her short life, love that we couldn't provide. So maybe one lesson of her life is to keep loving others and doing for others, even though we can no longer be with her.

Chapter 29

Since Lil has died, I've been haunted by my inability to recreate her unique voice in my head. With some people, I can easily have imaginary conversations with them because I know what they would say in different situations.

But she had such an original way of looking at things that I could never guess what would come out of her mouth. I asked her friends to send me anecdotes and little memories and that's helped me to keep her voice alive inside of me.

For instance, her friend Jeff sent:

> The first time me and Lil hung out just the two of us was when I offered to drive her to theater. On the way there Lillian was telling me how much she really wanted a "gay friend." Then she said, "Jeff....how do you feel about guys?"

I was so grateful to Jeff for sending it. It was so typical of her style, letting someone follow the way her mind was going and then making them laugh with a sudden twist at the end. I could perfectly imagine her saying it, the gleam in her eye, and then the smile growing as she waited for him to get it.

I found a last tape in the video camera. It had been started in March 2007, almost two years ago. We had always joked about how bad we were about recording family events, that it would seem like all we ever did was celebrate birthday parties and Christmas and go to softball games and school music concerts. But it had never really mattered before. Now, I wish that I had recorded everything.

I plugged the camera into the DVD recorder and Cate and I watched; it was the first time I had heard Lil's voice in more than a month.

The final sequence was taken right after her graduation from high school. She didn't want to have a party, but we had some friends over for dinner before she went out that night. It had been a beautiful summer evening and we were all sitting on the deck, surrounding her. Fortunately, I had kept the camera on for a long time when she gave a toast, and then while other people talked to her.

She always had such a lively face and it was beautiful to see how different emotions played across it as she talked. This openness was one of the things that made her so captivating and such a good actress. As she thought of different things she wanted to say, her face changed from smiling to frowning to joking, all in an instant. Her mind was so quick that she would constantly take delight in where it lead her, as if she were hearing her own words for the first time, the same as everyone else.

She looked tired in the video after having finished a long, demanding year of school. But she was poised and gracious as she thanked everyone for their support and love.

Annie said that Lil was her hero for the way she never complained about things, including her eyesight.

Lil thanked her, but then she looked down for awhile without saying anything. After a moment, a little smile appeared on her face as if she had some thought that amused her but she didn't want to share. I like to think that she was feeling proud of herself for all she had done, and love for all the people around her who were so excited for her and her future. A future that seemed so bright and limitless.

The Next Empty Thing

Dear God,
Let me live with my altar hollow,
the kind of nothing that

talks about Lillian's body
out there
in the box

With no need
for one more glimpse
because one more

glimpse would be
just that –
nothing more.

Let the box and its contents
roll over into
that next empty thing.

She is now
what she always was
and always will be

far removed from sweet flesh

below earth's edge, and the image

in the yellow-framed picture.

She, with no script in hand

moves through us

She, the perfect actress

her words

confetti, tossed high

in the air.

Let Lillian be

her story, her story

enough.

Cate Chason

Epilogue

Nearly ten years have gone by since Lillian's illness and death. I still calibrate all time in relation to those four weeks. If you ask me about a past event, my first thought will be to consider whether it was before or after Lil died.

After we got home, we still felt immense gratitude to the people at UNC hospital who had taken such good care of her, especially Dr. Charles. We couldn't imagine how much harder it would have been if we didn't have faith in the people who took care of her. But we felt like we had to do something about the poor care she got from the college health services. If she had been admitted to the hospital when she first complained of not being able to breathe, she might have been able to survive. Amazingly, experts we consulted said the doctor had met the standard of care even if we didn't think so.

We had a mediation with UNC in September 2011, two years after she had started school there. It helped when the university representatives started off by saying her death was a tragedy. They wanted to find ways to prevent something like this from happening again. Unfortunately, re-opening an infirmary where sick students could be cared for was not possible. But they instituted rules that would require the Campus Health Services to follow-up with students personally to make sure they were not getting worse. Students would no longer be told to go back to their dorms and not return. They would also coordinate with the disability services to make sure that sick students with disabilities got the services they needed.

To honor her memory, the university started a Lillian Chason Scholarship for undergraduates with an interest in dramatic arts. In addition, the Lillian Chason Undergraduate Excellence Fund is devoted to making enhancements to the undergraduate program. Near the beginning of each academic year, the Excellence Fund supports the production of a play that gives opportunities for undergraduates to participate, including freshmen. The director is recruited from the Brown/Trinity MFA theater program to increase the connection between the two institutions. None of the current students knew Lil personally, but Prof. David Navalinsky tirelessly works to make sure the students involved know her story. Every year, we go to Chapel Hill to see the play and meet the wonderful young people who, like Lil, love the theater.

Hannah went back to school and finished college with a psychology degree. After working for a few years, she realized she really did want to pursue medicine. This spring, she graduated from med school and is now doing a residency in emergency medicine.

Cate is still practicing acupuncture, less than full-time now. Nevertheless, she remains one of the most active, stimulating people I know. We added a small studio to the house so she could pursue her first love of painting. Even though she had not painted in 35 years, she fell back into it immediately and has created a beautiful collection of paintings and drawings. She gardens obsessively in the warm months and goes on long daily walks with her dog.

A few years ago, a doctor from the med school at Brown asked her to share her poems with students in the Gold's Humanism program. Eventually, she put them into a book called "Poems for Medical Students". She meets with the group once a year, where they read their favorites and ask her about their meaning. It is an emotional but fulfilling evening that gives these almost-doctors a chance to see illness and grief from a family's perspective.

I'm still teaching and doing research but I will never be the person I was. There will always be a hole in my life that may be covered over but can't be filled. With Lil's passing, I lost the illusion that life made sense, that we can count on anything. If it wasn't for wanting to be there for Hannah and Cate, I'm not sure what would have kept me going.

Days pass no matter how we feel about them, so here I am. I think of Lil often and would love to know what she would have to say about the state of the world. I'm sure it would be good.

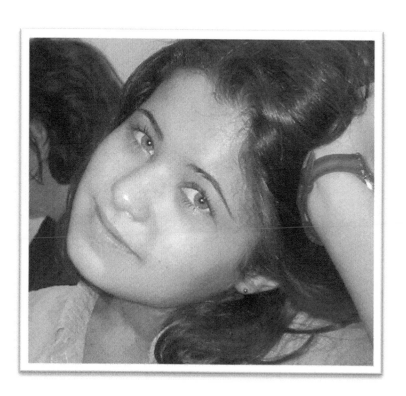

Acknowledgments

We are eternally grateful to the many doctors and staff at the UNC hospital who cared for Lil, especially to the amazing Dr. Anthony Gbollie Charles. We were helped by friends and family members in innumerable ways, back home and in Chapel Hill: sending cookies and cards, lending us their car, caring for the dogs, listening to us, teaching my class, reaching out to our mothers ... The support and love we received while we were at the hospital allowed us to keep our focus on Lil, and we are very thankful for that.

It is impossible to make a complete list of people to thank, but I want to acknowledge Melinda Ruley, Leslie Kreizmann and Marvin Saltzmann, Chuck and Kathie Sherman, Matt Gamache, Mark and Azadeh Perry, Joseph Megel, Pat and David Lea, Ruth Little and Britten Upchurch, Dorita Boyd, Barbara Gannon, Mary Pires, Nanda Gosh, Thom Jones, Charise Greene, Sandra and Ken Lambert, Julie Wilson and Martin Miner, Nancy and the other staff at the Ronald Macdonald House, my brother March Chason and my colleagues at Brown. The virtual community that developed through the Prayers for Lillian Facebook page opened our eyes to how many people cared about her.

This book began as a journal that I started in the hospital. But after Lillian's death, it became important to talk about more than just her illness, to let people know who Lillian was. The act of writing was a glorious way to stay connected with Lillian, a reason to bring up old memories and recall them in detail. This process was helped greatly by friends and members of writing groups whose suggestions helped me shape these stories into a coherent narrative. I want to thank Lorraine Keeney, Amy Tomasi, Robin Macausland and especially Rick Gamache for their positive thoughts and insightful comments.

Without Mark Perry, it is likely the manuscript would have just sat on my computer. He encouraged me and provided a path to publishing it. This has been like lightning striking twice since he is the same person who started the Facebook page that let others share her story. I thank Phyllis Ring for being a supportive editor. David Winsor patiently and tirelessly worked with us to develop the cover art.

Most of all, I want to thank my incredible wife Cate and daughter Hannah. It was a gift that we could be together in the hospital during this ordeal. Sharing my world with them, and Lillian, has been the joy of my life.